Volume 36, Issue 1, February 2009

Transfusion Medicine and Hemotherapy

Founded in 1973 as «Die Infusionstherapie» by H. Reissigl, H. Grobecker, U. Henneberg, K.H. Bäßler
Continued by: H.-D. Viering (1973–1977), A. Grünert (1982–1992), G. Kleinberger (1982–1988), K. Widhalm (1988–1992), G. Wolfram (1990–1992), J. Eckart (1992–1997), H. Forst (1992–1997), K. Meßmer (1992–1997), K. Peter (1992–1997), K.H. Usadel (1992–1997), B. Zwißler (1995–1997), K. Gutensohn (1998–2001), V. Kretschmer (1990–2002), W. Stangel (1992–2005), W. Dzik (1998–2005), H.G. Klein (1998–2005)

Official Organ of
German Society of Transfusion Medicine and Immunohematology

Deutsche Gesellschaft für
Transfusionsmedizin und
Immunhämatologie

DGTI

KARGER
Basel · Freiburg · Paris · London · New York ·
Bangalore · Bangkok · Singapore · Shanghai · Tokyo · Sydney

Transfusion Medicine
and Hemotherapy

Contents · Inhalt

Vol. 36, Issue 1, February 2009

KARGER

Fax +49 761 4 52 07 14
Information@Karger.de
www.karger.com

Accessible online at:
www.karger.com/tmh

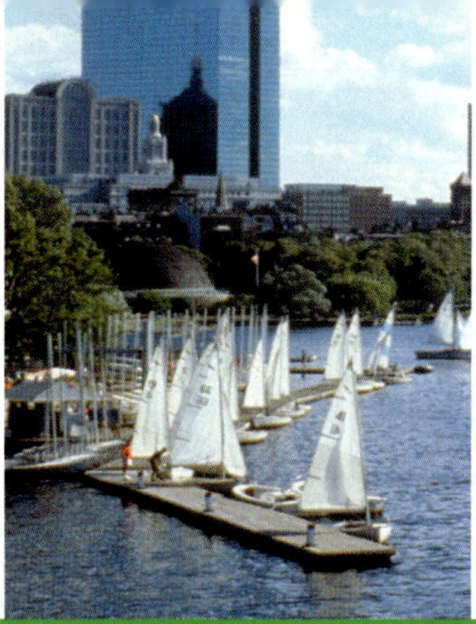

XXII Congress

The International Society on Thrombosis and Haemostasis

BOSTON 2009

July 11-16

International Society on Thrombosis and Haemostasis

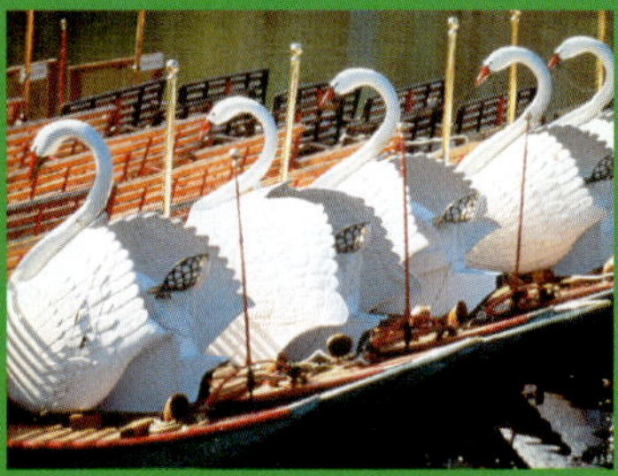

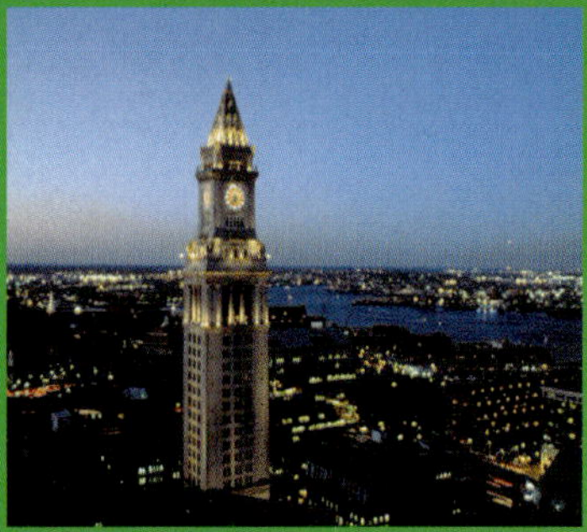

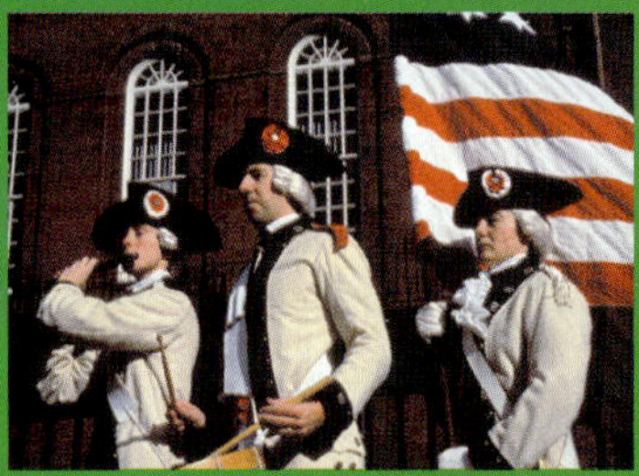

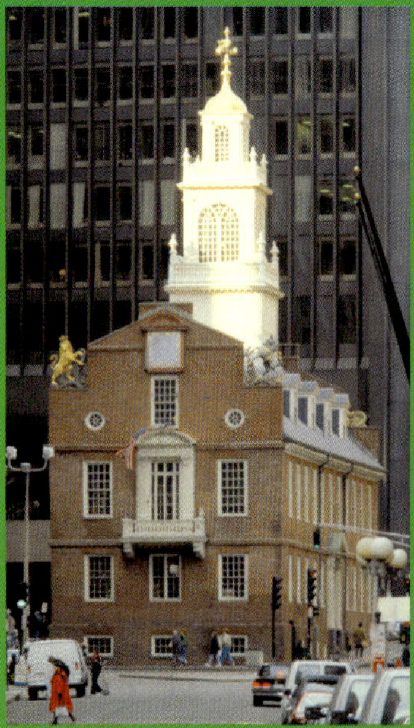

Important Dates and Deadlines

February 6, 2009
Abstract submission deadline

February 28, 2009
Early registration deadline

March 30, 2009
Notification of acceptance of abstracts

May 6, 2009
Accommodation reservation deadline

July 11-16, 2009
ISTH 2009

Email:
isth2009@mci-group.com
www.isth2009.com

PLENARY LECTURES

Thromboprophylaxis as a key patient safety priority: current approaches and future directions
Heparin-induced thrombocytopenia
Cardiovascular genetics
Contibution of allosteric disulfide bonds to regulation of hemostasis
Modern concepts of platelet activation during thrombus development
Stem cells, pluripotency, and nuclear reprogramming
von Willebrand assembly and secretion

STATE OF ART LECTURES

VASCULAR BIOLOGY
Inflammation and Atherosclerosis: Novel Targets for Plaque Progression and Regression
Endothelial and Vascular Cell Signaling
Endothelial Progenitor Cell Biology
Cues to Create a Mature Vasculature

HEMORRHAGIC DISORDERS
Von Willebrand Disease New Developments
Factor XI Revisited
Burning Questions in Hemophilia Inhibitors
Acquired Bleeding Disorders

COAGULATION AND FIBRINOLYSIS
Inflammation and Coagulation
Blood Coagulation-Systemic Effects in vivo
Fibrinogen/Fibrinolysis in the Brain
Novel Regulatory Reactions in Coagulation

PLATELETS (BASIC)
Novel Approaches to Understanding Hemostasis
Platelet Activation
Integrin Biology
Platelet Physiology/Pathophysiology

PLATELETS (CLINICAL)
Thrombopoietin Receptor Agonists
Immune Thrombocytopenia
Platelet Inhibition
Inherited Platelet Disorders

THROMBOTIC DISORDERS
Anticoagulation Duration after Idiopathic Venous Thrombosis - the Swinging Pendulum
Genomics and Vascular Disease: What Have We Learned About Thrombosis?
Pulmonary Embolism, 2009
Inflammation and Atherosclerosis: A Paradigm Shift?

ABSTRACT SYMPOSIA LECTURES

VASCULAR BIOLOGY
Signal Transduction in Vascular Cells
Regulation of Gene Expression in Vascular Cells
Shear Stress, Rheology, and Mechanical Signaling Responses
Inflammation
Blood Vessel Development
Inflammation and Vascular Pathobiology
Atherosclerosis

HEMORRHAGIC DISORDERS
Factor VIII and VWF
Hemophilia and Rare Blood Disorders
Women and Bleeding Disorders
New Products in Hemophilia and vWD
von Willebrand disease
Neonatal/Pediatric Hemostasis
Intracranial Hemorrhage
Update on gene therapy

COAGULATION AND FIBRINOLYSIS
Extrinsic Pathway of Coagulation
Intrinsic Pathway of Coagulation
Contact Pathway
Cofactors
Serpins/Inhibitors
Protease Structure/Function
Fibrinogen/Fibrinolysis
Regulation of Coagulation

PLATELETS (BASIC)
Phosphatases and Platelet Activation
Platelet Biochemistry and Biology
Adhesion and Cohesion
Novel Approaches to Understanding Platelet Biolc
Platelets and Systemic Disorders
Megakaryocytes and Thrombopoiesis
Polymorphisms, Heterogeneity and the Mechanisr of Platelet Disorders
ADAMTS13, TTP and Related Disorders
Platelets as Drug Targets

PLATELETS (CLINICAL)
Immunology and Treatment of ITP
Pathophysiology of HIT
TTP & ADAMTS13
Platelet Function Tests
Platelets and Myeloproliferative Syndromes
Platelet Transfusion
Microparticles
Platelets and Cancer

THROMBOTIC DISORDERS
Indications for Thrombophilia Testing in Asymptomatic Family Members
Long-Term Complications of VTE: Epidemiology, Prevention and Treatment/Post-Thrombotic Syndrome
Estrogens and Vascular Disease: Non-Oral Postmenopausal Hormones and Risk of Thromb
Best Use of Vena Cava Filters
Thrombolysis of Lower Extremity DVT
Paradoxical Embolus and Treatment of PFO
Pathogenesis of Pre-Eclampsia
Neonatal Stroke

Transfusion Medicine and Hemotherapy

Editorial

Transfus Med Hemother 2009;36:5–6
DOI: 10.1159/000184685

Still in Focus: Assessment of Blood-Borne Pathogens

Rainer Seitz[a] Margarethe Heiden[a] Ruth Offergeld[b] Reinhard Burger[b]

[a] Paul-Ehrlich-Institut, Langen,
[b] Robert Koch-Institut, Berlin, Germany

The German Advisory Committee Blood (Arbeitskreis Blut) was installed by the German Federal Ministry of Health 15 years ago, under the impression of an epidemic of virus transmissions through blood products. The task of this committee, which is based at the Robert Koch-Institut in Berlin, is to provide reliable scientific advice to the government concerning the quality and safety as well as the appropriate use of blood and blood products. The status of the Arbeitskreis Blut has been enhanced by stipulating its role and operation in the German Transfusion Act of 1998. All the time since its foundation, a major focus of work has been the safety regarding transmission of infectious agents. The Arbeitskreis Blut established a permanent subgroup 'Assessment of Pathogens Transmissible by Blood', meeting regularly at the Paul-Ehrlich-Institut in Langen, dedicated to compiling and updating information on infectious agents transmitted by blood.

In the past decades, the safety of blood and blood products has increased dramatically and is meanwhile very high. This impressive improvement of pathogen safety is due to well established donor criteria and advancements of technology leading to extremely sensitive and specific tests used for donor screening. The serological testing, i.e. the per se already very efficient detection of antibodies or antigens, has been supplemented by the introduction of nucleic acid amplification technology (NAT) for HCV genome in 1999, and for HIV genome in 2004. The success of this strategy is demonstrated by haemovigilance data collected by the Paul-Ehrlich-Institut: Since the introduction of NAT, only one single case of HCV and one single case of HIV transmission by blood components have been reported in Germany, where about 4.5 million whole blood donations take place annually. Ongoing projects aim at increasing the safety margin of blood components even further by pathogen inactivation procedures. Effective virus inactivation steps became mandatory for plasma derivatives about 20 years ago and practically eliminated the transmission of viral diseases by these products. This success story helped very much to restore the confidence of patients into blood products. However, unfortunately a 'zero risk' cannot be reached with biological products. As a matter of fact, pathogens are a moving target, and there is a continuous race between progress of science and technology and emerging or re-emerging pathogens. New agents may pose particular risks because they may escape the established screening systems, and it may be difficult to develop test methods suitable for donor screening, as in the case of the agent causing variant Creutzfeldt-Jakob disease (vCJD). 'Old' pathogens may re-emerge due to mutations, changes in their habitat and influence of human lifestyle, particularly the ever-growing international travel; recent examples may be found among arthropod-borne viruses, bacteria and parasites for example.

Thus, there is no reason to lay back in complacency, and the Arbeitskreis Blut subgroup 'Assessment of Pathogens Transmissible by Blood' is continuing its work in order to provide timely advice. All reviews have been published in Transfusion Medicine And Hemotherapy as soon as they were finalised. The frequent request from e.g. transfusionists, scientific societies and regulators to provide these assessments, which are focused strongly on the perspective for blood product safety, in a single issue of a journal or booklet in order to have the relevant information ready at hand has been met already with a special issue in August 2005 [1]. The present issue of Transfusion Medicine And Hemotherapy provides additional papers on Influenza [2], Hepatitis E [3], Malaria [4], and Arbobacteria [5], and the paper on Arboparasites [6] published in the present issue in its English version for the first time.

With the task to develop a strategy for a save blood supply in view of the variant Creutzfeldt-Jakob disease (vCJD), an expert working group was appointed by the German Federal Minister of Health in 2001. A comprehensive report of this group has been published in Transfusion Medicine And Hemotherapy in 2006 [7]. Of particular concern are reports in

KARGER

Fax +49 761 4 52 07 14
Information@Karger.de
www.karger.com

Accessible online at:
www.karger.com/tmh

Prof. Dr. med. Rainer Seitz
Paul-Ehrlich-Institut
Paul-Ehrlich-Straße 51–59, 63225 Langen (Germany)
Tel. +49 6103 77–26 01, Fax -1250
E-mail seira@pei.de

the past years of obvious transmission of the vCJD agent by transfusion of red cells, which raises the issue of donor screening. The current status of epidemiology, the scientific background of vCJD diagnostics, the numerous recent developments towards test systems as well as regulatory aspects and ethical problems were extensively discussed by the expert group; the English version of the report is published in the present issue [8].

The Arbeitskreis Blut recognizes and acknowledges the work done by both groups in the preparation of the comprehensive statements. Also the excellent secretarial support by Mrs. Knoess, Mrs. Taylor, and Mrs. Erikli is gratefully appreciated. We are confident that the present special issue of TRANSFUSION MEDICINE AND HEMOTHERAPY provides another helpful reference manual for rapid and reliable information on relevant blood-borne agents, and strategic considerations to ensure a safe blood supply.

References

1 Assessment of Pathogens Transmissible By Blood: Statements of the German `National Advisory Committee Blood` (Arbeitskreis Blut). Transfus Med Hemother 2005;32(3/4):105–240.
2 Arbeitskreis Blut, Untergruppe «Bewertung Blutassoziierter Krankheitserreger»: Influenza Virus. Transfus Med Hemother 2008;35(5):42–49.
3 Arbeitskreis Blut, Untergruppe «Bewertung Blutassoziierter Krankheitserreger»: Hepatitis E Virus. Transfus Med Hemother 2008;35(5):50–57.
4 Arbeitskreis Blut, Untergruppe «Bewertung Blutassoziierter Krankheitserreger»: Malaria. Transfus Med Hemother 2008;35(5):122–134.
5 Arbeitskreis Blut, Untergruppe «Bewertung Blutassoziierter Krankheitserreger»: Arbobacteria – pathogens transmittable by arthropods. Transfus Med Hemother 2008;35(5):374–390
6 Arbeitskreis Blut, Untergruppe «Bewertung Blutassoziierter Krankheitserreger»: Arboprotozoae. Transfus Med Hemother 2009;35(1):8–31.
7 Overall Blood Supply with Regard to Variant Creutzfeldt-Jakob Disease (vCJD): Report of the Working Group Commissioned by the German Federal Ministry of Health, April 13, 2006. Transf Med Hemother 2006;33(suppl. 2):VII + 40.
8 Working Group 'Overall Blood Supply Strategy with Regard to Variant Creutzfeldt-Jakob Disease (vCJD)': Statement on the development and implementation of test systems suitable for the screening of blood donors for variant Creutzfeldt-Jakob disease. Transfus Med Hemother 2009;35(1):79–93.

Transfusion Medicine and Hemotherapy

Transfus Med Hemother 2009;36:8–31
DOI: 10.1159/000187642

Arboprotozoae

Arbeitskreis Blut, Untergruppe «Bewertung Blutassoziierter Krankheitserreger»

Arboprotozoae represent protozoal infectious agents transmissible by arthropods. This paper only deals with arboprotozoae which can be transmitted by blood transfusion in an epidemiologically relevant way. Essential characteristics and possible transmissibility are described for the following arboprotozoae:

A *Leishmania*
B *Trypanosoma brucei gambiense* and *rhodesiense, Trypanosoma cruzi*
C *Babesia microti* and/or *divergens*
D *Toxoplasma gondii*

Plasmodium sp. was described previously [1].

Infectious agents such as *Giardia lamblia, Dientamoeba* sp., *Entamoeba* sp., *Cryptosporidium parvum* and *Isospora belli* are also protozoae which can infect humans, depending on region, food and water hygiene, and which can be transmitted via blood in exceptional cases [2]. They cause infections of the gastrointestinal tract and occasionally lead to penetration of tissue layers so that they are also present in the blood following phagocytosis by macrophages/monocytes within a short period, e.g. in only few days up to a week. After the gastrointestinal symptoms have subsided, these agents are normally no longer present in the blood. Up to now, transmissions by these protozoae have not been reported in Germany. Therefore, they will not be discussed in detail. Since acutely infected donors are excluded from donating blood for 4 weeks following an episode of diarrhoea, the probability of an infection is negligibly low. However, such a transmission cannot be ruled out entirely as reports of transmissions by organs and stem cells show [3].

The three typical clinical patterns of malaria and the transmission of the four types of plasmodia (*Plasmodium falciparum, Plasmodium ovale, Plasmodium vivax* and *Plasmodium malariae*) by blood have already been described by the subgroup of the Advisory Committee Blood (Arbeitskreis Blut) [1] and are therefore not discussed in more detail in this paper. Plasmodia have adapted to humans in such a way that they cannot be transmitted from humans to different species (the chimpanzee is a rare exception) and vice versa. Therefore – unlike the pathogens discussed here – they are not zoonoses.

The protozoae listed in table 1 are also wide-spread in animals. They are by definition typical pathogenic agents of zoonoses and can therefore not be eradicated. The transmission risk can normally be reduced by keeping apart and combating the vector or vehicle. Attempts at developing a protective vaccine against these protozoae have so far not been successful and will prove to be difficult in future, too, due to the great variability of the surface antigens of the protozoae. In this context, transmission of a protozoa infection by domestic animals, with the exception of malaria, as explained above, should also be considered.

A *Leishmania* spp.

A 1 Current Knowledge about the Pathogen

These protozoae were characterised by Leishman and Donovan in 1903. Leishmania is wide-spread in tropical and subtropical regions world-wide. Indications pointing to mutilating infections of the face can be found on ceramic containers excavated in Central America that date as far back as 1,000 years, and on pictures of the Spanish conquerors in the 16th century [4]. In 1911, Gaspar Vianna found the difference in the replication cycles between *Leishmania* of the Old World and that of the New World. Leishmaniasis of the Old World was described around 1500 AD [4] in the region of present-day Afghanistan in the Middle East. The *Leishmania* pathogen was described for the first time by the Russian military doctor Borovsky in a skin wound in 1898 [5].

Leishmania belongs to the family of trypanosomatides in the order of kinetoplastides, and their evolution probably dates back 1 billion years.

KARGER

Fax +49 761 4 52 07 14
Information@Karger.de
www.karger.com

Accessible online at:
www.karger.com/tmh

Prof. Dr. med. Rainer Seitz
Paul-Ehrlich-Institut
Paul-Ehrlich-Straße 51–59, 63225 Langen (Germany)
Tel. +49 6103 77-2601, Fax -1250
E-mail seira@pei.de

Table 1. Protozoal infectious agents: Route of transmission, symptoms, and geographical distribution

Section	Protozoon	Route of transmission/vector	Symptoms	Duration of disease	Geographical distribution
A	*Leishmania* sp. *Viannia*	sand fly (*Phlebotomus* and *Lutzomyia*), horse fly (*Tabanidae*), tick (*Ornithodorus*)	cutaneous mucocutaneous visceral	3 weeks up to life-long	Near East Mediterranean Central Asia South Asia Central America South America Central Africa
B	*Trypanosoma cruzi*	kissing bugs, e.g. *Triatoma, Rhonius, Panstrongylus* via the faeces	Chagas disease	1 week up to life-long	Latin America South America
B	*Trypanosoma brucei*	tsetse fly (*Glossina morsitans*)	sleeping sickness	3 weeks up to 3 years for *T. brucei gambiense* and 3 weeks up to 20 years for *T. brucei rhodesiense*	West Africa East Africa
C	*Babesia* sp.	tick (*Ixodes ricinus, Ornithodorus, Dermatocentor, Amblyomma*	babesiosis	approximately 4 weeks up to several years	Europe North America, there, it particularly infects cattle
	Plasmodium	anopheles mosquito	tropical malaria tertian malaria quartan malaria	seldom 11, usually 17 days up to decades, depending on the *Plasmodium* species	tropical zone [cf. 1]
D	*Toxoplasma gondii*	infection by smearing, via cat faeces, contaminated vegetables, animal hair, e.g. cat hair or raw meet. Seldom also transmission via arthropods, e.g. cockroach or fly, by contact with open wounds of the skin and the mucosae	toxoplasmosis	approximately 3 weeks, in cysts (bradyzoites), remains infectious over decades. Only short phase of spreading in blood	world-wide

Approximately 350 million people are threatened by *Leishmania* [6], and around 12 million have chronic pathological symptoms. Around 90% of all cases of visceral leishmaniasis occur in eastern India and Bangladesh, in Sudan and in Brazil. Around 90% of the cases of cutaneous leishmaniasis occur in the countries of the Middle East, in Afghanistan up to Central Asia, and in Latin America up to Peru, and around 90% of the cases of mucocutaneous leishmaniasis in Brazil, Bolivia and Peru.
The genus Leishmania is subdivided into the subgenera *Leishmania* (world-wide geographical distribution) and *Viannia* (only occurs in America). *Viannia's* replication cycle slightly differs in the vector. The classification of *Leishmania* has not yet been completed. Different *Leishmania* types can cause clinically overlapping clinical symptoms. Important *Leishmania* species include: *L. donovani, L. infantum, L. major, L. chagasi, L. amazonensis, L. brasiliana, L. mexicana, L. peruviana* and others.

A 1.1 Characteristics of Leishmania *spp.*

In dependency of the replication organ or host, diploid *Leishmania* have a flagellum (promastigotes) or lack the flagellum (amastigotes), e.g. when growing in the cells of a reticuloendothelial system of mammals. *Leishmania* actively penetrate the cell wall and replicate there. They are taken up into the vector during the blood-sucking process of sand flies of the *Phlebotomus* species in Europe and Asia, and of the *Lutzomyia* species in the two Americas [7]. There, they replicate in the intestines and accumulate in the foregut. Then, they are injected into the skin of the mammal by the sting.

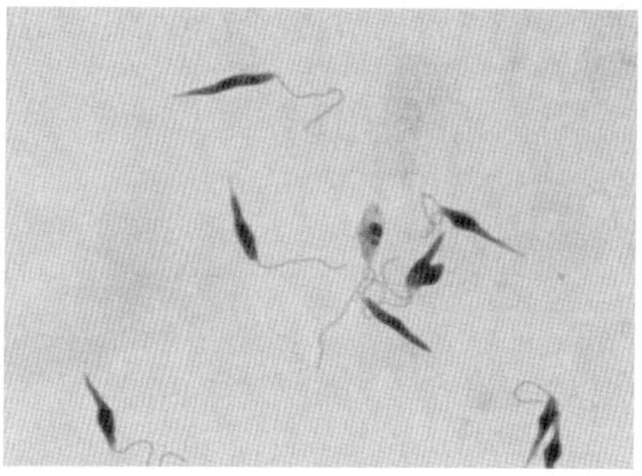

Fig. 1. *Leishmania.* Promastigotes with polar flagellum, Tricon stain. Original preparation from the Tropeninstitut (Institute for Tropical Medicine) of the Ludwig-Maximilians-University, Munich, Prof. Löscher.

A 1.1.1 Structure

Leishmania have a length of 2–3 µm and a width of 0.7–1 µm. As promastigotes, they have a polar flagellum of 2–3 µm in length when they are in the vector (fig. 1). They change into the

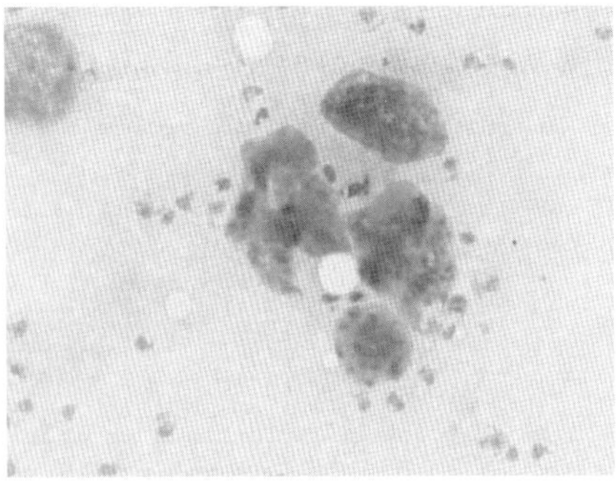

Fig. 2. *Leishmania.* Amastigotes without flagellum, Tricon stain. Original preparation from the Tropeninstitut (Institute for Tropical Medicine) of the Ludwig-Maximilians-University, Munich, Prof. Löscher.

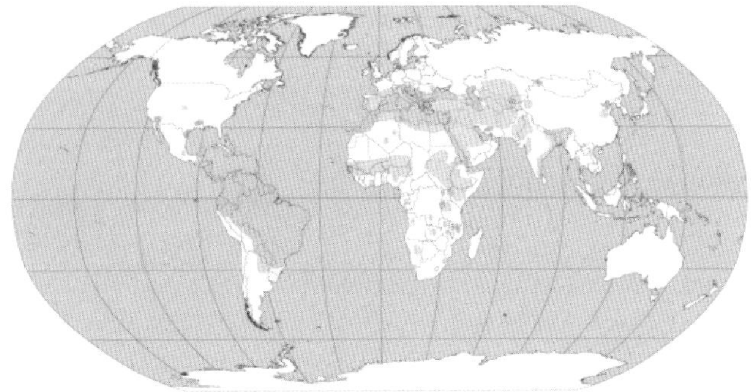

Fig. 3. World-wide distribution of *Leishmania* spp., derived from the information generally accessible in 2008.

elongated to round amastigotes (3–5 μm) that lack the flagellum when they are in human macrophages or other cells (fig. 2). The cell body shows a large core and a kinetoplast. The flagellum of amastigotes remains in the cell membrane. *Leishmania* can be stained by trichrome-, Giemsa- and haematoxylin-eosin staining.

A 1.1.2 Replication

A sexual replication phase has so far not been described for *Leishmania*. In humans, *Leishmania* replicates in macrophages or other mononuclear cells, in Langerhans and dendritic cells of the skin or in Kupffer cells of the liver within the acidic parasitophorous vacuole after an incubation period of approximately 10 days. Cell death causes amastigotes to be released which infect further cells.

A 1.2 Infection and Infectious Disease

Visceral leishmaniasis, synonym: kala-azar: After a sand fly sting, the promastigotes are ingested by macrophages and replicate in an intracellular manner. A papule remains visible at the stinging site which swells up due to the entering leucocytes. The pathogens propagate from the stinging site causing lymphadenopathy and progressive swelling of the spleen and liver. Depending on the immune response, the infection is either overcome or results in chronic illness or fatal outcome.

Cutaneous leishmaniasis: Typical clinical manifestations include the oriental sore or aleppo button in the Near East and the cutaneous verruciform leishmaniasis in South America. After the sting, the amastigotes replicate within the Langerhans cells of the skin. Following this, leucocytes enter the site, the peripheral wall of the site swells up and a papule forms, and finally, after weeks, an ulcer with white base. The lesions partly resemble lepra. After the ulcer has healed, relapses can occur since amastigotes persist in some cells and can be released sporadically. Infected individuals show persistent fever, weight loss, fatigue, exhaustion, and hepatosplenomegaly. Laboratory tests reveal anaemia, leucopenia, and hypergammaglobulinaemia.

A 1.3 Epidemiology

Leishmania is wide-spread in the subtropical regions of the world where the main vector, the sand fly (*Phlebotomus* and *Lutzomyia*), is located as well as habitats for its replication, such as suitable wild and productive livestock reservoirs (fig. 3). Poor hygienic conditions also contribute to the spreading of the vector. Apart from being transmitted by the vectors sand fly, horse fly and tick, *Leishmania* can also be transmitted parenterally by blood transfusion, needle prick lesions and intravenous (i.v.) drug consumption.

L. donovani is wide-spread in Eastern India, Bangladesh, East Africa (particularly Sudan and Kenya) and in the entire Mediterranean region, and leads to the visceral form of leishmaniasis (kala-azar). In case of chronic courses, especially if the primary infection occurs in a child, the skin is also affected, and the vectors are infected during the sting and the subsequent blood uptake. Animal reservoirs include cattle, dog, cat, rat, mouse and small domestic animals. The *Leishmania aethiopica* infection is similar to that of *L. donovani*. Double infections have been described with various *Leishmania* species.

In the Gulf region of the Arabian world, US soldiers became infected with *Leishmania tropica* during the Gulf War [8]. Infections of soldiers from Iraq and Afghanistan are known [9]. No *Leishmania* transmissions by blood transfusions have so far been reported in Germany.

In the rural regions of Brazil, *L. infantum/L. chagasi* has caused regionally restricted epidemics. *L. peruviana* more frequently caused the cutaneous form of leishmaniasis such as *L. mexicana*, *amazonensis*, and *brasiliensis*, which rank among the more wide-spread species in that region. *L. brasiliensis* also causes the mucocutaneous form, called espundia. It causes inflammations and ulcers which may persist up to 6 years.

Visceral leishmaniasis has been observed in patients with the immune deficiency HIV in Switzerland [10] and in some patients in Spain [11]. Up to late 1995, 734 AIDS-infected patients were reported to the WHO from France, Italy, Portugal and Spain [33]. In addition, a high number of *Leishmania* and HIV-co-infected individuals are known from Brazil, Ethiopia and India from WHO studies [12].

A chronic infection was identified in Germany in one patient with erythaematous, infiltrative plaques [13], in 42 patients, who were examined between 2001 and 2004 [14] and in 58 patients in the Berlin area between 2000 and 2002 [15]. Out of the 58 patients in the Berlin area, 48 were Germans who had acquired their infection as tourists in the following countries: in Europe (France, Italy, Malta and Spain), in America (Brazil, Bolivia, Ecuador, French Guyana and Peru), in Asia (Afghanistan, United Arabian Emirates, Syria and Turkey), and in Africa (Egypt, Kenya and Libya). The data show that *Leishmania* also exists in Germany, but endogenous transmissions have so far not been described in Germany. In one case of visceral leishmaniasis in a child which had not stayed in an endemic region, *Leishmania* transmission in Germany cannot be ruled out [16]. In 130 imported *Leishmania* infections in Germany, the average time from occurrence of the symptoms up to diagnosis was 3–4 months [17].

A 1.4 Detection Methods and Their Significance

A 1.4.1 Identification of the Pathogen

a) Microscopy: Amastigotes (fig. 2) can be detected in tissue, squash specimens of the ulcer, enriched mononuclear cells of the blood and bone marrow cells.
b) Culture: *Leishmania* can be cultured from tissue in Novy, Mac Neal, and Nicoll medium (NNN) [18]. Isolation is performed from peripheral blood mononuclear cells (PBMC) which are enriched via gradient centrifugation from blood and kept in culture for several months [19].
c) NAT (nucleic acid testing): Kinetoplast DNA from PBMC is used for identification in blood [20]. For this purpose, a duplex PCR was developed [21] or a real-time PCR adapted [22, 23]. A sensitivity level of 1 parasite per 8 µl blood can be reached, while parasitaemia levels may fluctuate between 32 and 188,000 parasites/ml blood [22].

Leishmania can also be identified via the DNA of the glucose-6-phosphate dehydrogenase of the pathogen [24]. This test is particularly suitable for the identification of the *Viannia* species which circulate in Brazil.

A real-time PCR was developed which is located in the cytochrome b-gene of *Leishmania* and with which *Leishmania* species can be identified at the same time [25].

A PCR which amplifies ‘minicircles' in kinetoplasts and simultaneously permits assignment of the *Leishmania* species by geographical regions was described in 2008 [26]. Sensitivity levels of the test were 5 parasites/ml blood.

A 1.4.2 Detection of Antibodies

The detection of antibodies means there is an immunological response to *Leishmania*. It does not automatically mean that the disease has been overcome.

a) ELISA is available both as commercial and as in-house test with a sensitivity of around 93%. False-positive results can occur due to cross-reactivity of antibodies against *Mycobacterium leprae* and *Trypanosoma* [27].
b) Western blot: Western blot strips can be produced in special laboratories with a reaction involving proteins with molecular weights of 40, 18, and 14.4 kDa having particular informative value [28, 20].

A 2 Blood and Plasma Donors

Cutaneous inoculation and manifestation of the primary infection can also lead to parasitaemia, as shown in mice.
Leishmania remains replication-competent up to 25 days after a blood sample was drawn. Replication-competent *Leishmania* can also be identified in red blood cell and platelet concentrates, but not in fresh frozen plasma (FFP) [8].

A 2.1 Prevalence and Incidence in Donor Populations

Out of 565 blood donors in South France, 76 were seropositive, and in 9 of these donors, *L. infantum* could be detected by means of PCR and culturing. This corresponds to a prevalence of 1.2%. This analysis shows that *L. infantum* with undulating parasitaemia can occur periodically in exposed but healthy seropositive blood donors [20].

A 2.2 Definition of Exclusion Criteria

The general guidelines of the Bundesärztekammer (German Medical Association) and the Paul-Ehrlich-Institut [29, 30] apply to the exclusion of potentially infectious donors.
So far, it has not been necessary to define specific exclusion criteria for the prevention of *Leishmania* transmission in Germany. A temporal deferral after a stay in endemic regions with sand fly exposure might be thinkable. A deferral of persons who stayed in *Leishmania*-endemic areas such as the Kosovo or Afghanistan for longer periods could also be considered.
In Spain, a country which is more affected by leishmaniasis than Germany, no further *Leishmania*-specific deferral criteria are used besides the deferral after travelling to malaria-, HTLV-1- and Chagas-endemic areas. Tests for *Leishmania* are not performed, since the compulsory leucocyte depletion used in Spain is considered as a suitable prevention measure. However, donors who stayed in an endemic region in Italy or Spain are deferred from donating blood for 6 months [31].

A 2.3 Donor Testing and Significance

A screening test for antibodies in donors of blood and blood components is currently not performed in Germany. As described in section A 1.4, sensitivity levels of around 93% are to be expected

for ELISA tests. The epidemiological situation of few annual *Leishmania* infections imported from endemic countries currently do not justify general testing for *Leishmania* antibodies.
The detection of *Leishmania* in blood by means of NAT is possible. Sensitivity levels of the NAT rise if mononuclear cells of the blood are used (cf. section A 1.4). Due to the epidemiological situation of only isolated cases of clinical manifestation among the normal population and the absence of documented cases of transmission by blood donation in Germany, no NAT tests are currently performed.

A 2.4 Donor Interviews

Donors are not interviewed after a stay in endemic regions or after stings of *Phlebotomus* in the Mediterranean region or *Lutzomyia* in Central and South America. However, they are excluded for 6 months after staying in regions were the occurrence of *Leishmania* and malaria overlap.

A 2.5 Donor Information and Counselling

No donor information regarding *Leishmania* and the possibility of *Leishmania* transmission nor advice on the clinical outcome and chronic course takes place.

A 3 Recipient

A 3.1 Prevalence and Incidence of Blood-Associated Infections and Infectious Diseases in Recipient Populations

No examinations are carried out on the prevalence and incidence of *Leishmania* in recipients of blood and blood products in Germany.

A 3.2 Immune Status (Resistance, Existing Immunity, Immune Response, Age, Exogenous Factors)

Leishmania can be transmitted even if the defence situation is good. In this case the infection can be partly overcome as described in section A 1.2. A clinically visible defence reaction can be expected after approximately 3 weeks. Particularly severe clinical outcomes are found in the case of an immune disorder, e.g. AIDS [32, 33].

A 3.3 Severity and Course of the Disease

As described in section A 1.2, the infection can be overcome spontaneously or take on the chronic form with cutaneous or visceral manifestation, depending on the inoculation dose, the *Leishmania* species, the initial defence reaction and the treatment performed. If left untreated, leishmaniasis can result in fatal outcome.

A 3.4 Therapy and Prophylaxis

Liposomal amphotericin B (Ambisome) has proved to be the treatment of choice in visceral leishmaniasis. It is administered weekly over a period of 4 weeks, in case of an immune disorder over a period of 6 weeks. In India, approximately 40% of the *Leishmania* types are resistant to pentavalent antimon. Miltefosin (Impavido) is a more recent, efficacious substance, which is also used against cutaneous leishmaniasis, and can be administered to out-patients [34]. The stinging site can be treated with 15% paromomycin and 12% methylbenzetoniumchloride after the ulcer has formed. Miltefosin is also a product which is used successfully in India for the treatment of visceral leishmaniasis [35].
Cutaneous leishmaniasis can also be treated successfully with a combination of imiquimod and megluminantimoniat [36]. Pentamidin, which is available as second-line medication, is eliminated from amastigotes via the ABC transporter [37]. Megluminantimoniat could be more efficacious if encapsulated by liposomes [38].
Three methods are available for preventing the disease:
- mechanical protection from the stinging attacks by the sand fly,
- eradication of the vector by insecticides in regions with particularly high infestation, and
- decontamination of the livestock and domestic animals by appropriate treatment or elimination of infected animals; checking of imported live animals, particularly dogs, from endemic areas.

Preventative medicinal products or vaccinations are not available.

A 3.5 Transmissibility

As described in section A 1.2, *Leishmania* can be infectious in the blood component up to 25 days after it was collected. Therefore, the agent can be transmitted via blood and blood products. Eleven transmissions by blood transfusion have been reported [39] and, in addition, 32 by haemodialysis in Brazil [40]. Transmission from human to human by social contacts has not been described. Known vectors include *Phlebotomus*, *Tabanides* and *Lutzomyia*.
The first laboratory infection probably occurred in China in 1930. The first proven laboratory infection with *L. donovani* was reported in 1950 [41]. Altogether, 12 laboratory transmissions with *Leishmania* have been published, out of which 6 occurred in the USA, 3 in Latin America, and 1 each in Asia, Canada and Europe [42]. More than half of the infections described occurred after parenteral inoculation. These transmissions are avoidable if the appropriate precautionary measures are observed.

A 3.6 Frequency of Administration, Type and Amount of Blood Products

Leishmania agents are enriched in leucocytes [43]. They can be transmitted by red blood cells, granulocytes and platelet concentrates. Because of the low prevalence and incidence in Germany, the type and quantity of the blood products are of no significance.

A 4 Blood Products

A 4.1 Infectious Load of the Starting Material and Test Methods

Leishmania can be transmitted by blood and blood products, which was proven in endemic regions [9, 20]. In one case described, transmission of the infection by blood from an asymptomatic carrier to a newborn led to fever and hepatosplenomegaly within 1 month and to the infant's death within 7 months [39]. Thrombocyte concentrates, too, can transmit *Leishmania*, which led to the visceral form, as shown in one report from India [44].

A 4.2 Methods for Removal and Inactivation of the Infectious Agent

Since *Leishmania* is cell-bound, all cell-containing contaminated blood products can transmit *Leishmania* [8]. Leucocyte depletion can reduce the burden by 3–4 $\log_{10}$ if carried out in a timely manner after the blood is drawn [43, 45].
When using sterile filtered plasma, *Leishmania* is without any significance since the pathogen is retained in the filter [43]. *Leishmania* agents are eliminated and/or inactivated during the fractionation of products such as plasma for the preparation of coagulation factors and immunoglobulin.
Leishmania can be inactivated by DNA intercalating photoinactivators such as thiopyrilium after light irradiation by more than 5.7 $\log_{10}$ $TCID_{50}$ [46]. Inactivation can also be carried out by treatment with psoralen and UV light, bringing about a reduction of 4 $\log_{10}$ [47], and riboflavin and UV light, in which case a reduction of approximately 5 $\log_{10}$ in plasma and platelet concentrates was achieved [48].
Leishmanias can be removed entirely by sterile filtration and do therefore not have any significance for plasma derivatives.

A 4.3 Feasibility and Validation of Procedures for Removal/ Inactivation of the Infectious Agent

After successful replication of *Leishmania* in culture media and cell culture as well as after identification and quantification of the agent via PCR, spike experiments by external contamination have become possible and have been carried out [43]. Filtration via leucocyte filter can reduce promastigotes in plasma by up to 6–8 $\log_{10}$; filtration of red blood cell concentrates brought about a reduction of up to 4 $\log_{10}$ after 2 weeks storage. The reduction of free promastigotes and amastigotes is explained by their negative surface charge and adsorption to the filter matrix [49].

A 5 Assessment

Persons who live in Germany are also infected with *Leishmania* when travelling to endemic regions after vector stings. The essential vectors of the Mediterranean (*Phlebotomus*) or American regions (*Lutzomyia*) were identified in Germany in isolated cases. However, currently the highly infected animal reservoir, by which the vector would be infected, is still missing. Individuals with chronic leishmaniasis are in any case permanently excluded from donation, due to their impaired state of health, partly with fever and anaemia. Donors in whom leishmaniasis has been detected, whether cutaneous or visceral, should be permanently excluded from donation [9, 50].
In Germany the risk of *Leishmania* transmission via blood is very low, and via plasmas products non-existent. Therefore, there is currently no justification for introducing testing, neither as an antibody test nor by NAT. Nevertheless, the epidemiological development regarding both the agent and the vector should be observed.

B ***Trypanosoma***

B 1 Current Knowledge about the Pathogen

Carlos Chagas described American trypanosomiasis in Brazil at the beginning of the 20th century [51]. He also identified the transmission mechanism of trypanosomes via kissing bugs, and transmitted trypanosomes from the blood of infected patients to guinea pigs and monkeys [52]. The pathogen was identified by Oswaldo Cruz. Around 18 million people are infected with Chagas disease [4].
African trypanosomiasis was first described by John Atkin in 1721 and then by Thomas Winterbottom in 1803 [4, 53]. In 1881, Griffith Evans found trypanosomes in the blood of horses and dromedaries infected with Surra disease, in 1894, David Bruce detected the pathogens during an outbreak of nagana disease in cattle in South Africa, and in 1891, Gustave Nepveu identified them in human blood of infected hunters [54].
The genus of *Trypanosoma* consists of 20 species out of which 2 or 3 are human pathogenic [55]. *Trypanosoma cruzi*, also known as *Schizotrypanum cruzi* has a geographical distribution ranging from Mexico up to Central Argentina and Chile, while *Trypanosoma brucei gambiense* prevails in West and Central Africa, and *Trypanosoma brucei rhodesiense* in East Africa. *T. cruzi* is transmitted by the kissing bug (*Triatoma infestans*) and

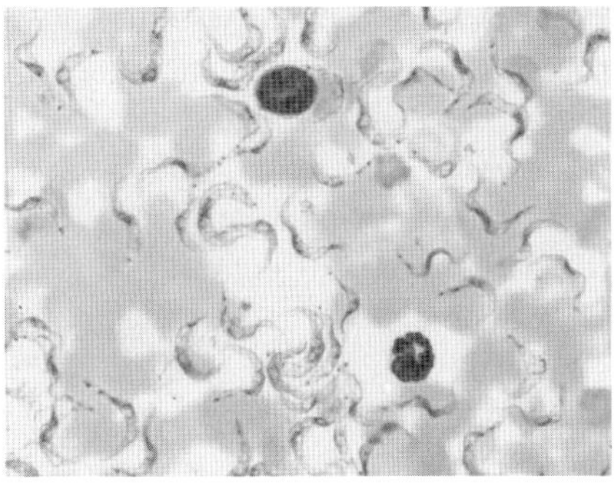

Fig. 4. Blood smear from a mouse infected with trypanosomas, May-Grünwald-Giemsa stain. In this picture, no distinction can be seen between *T. cruzi* and *T. brucei*. Preparation from the Friedrich-Löffler-Institut für Medizinische Mikrobiologie (Friedrich-Löffler-Institute for Medical Biology), University Hospital of Greifswald, Germany.

other bugs; *T. brucei* is transmitted by the tsetse fly. American trypanosomes cause Chagas disease while African trypanosomes cause sleeping sickness. Both diseases are zoonoses. The domestic animals armadillo and opossum and the invertebrates triatoma are the main hosts for *T. cruzi*. Hosts for *T. brucei* include wild animals such as antilopes, gazelles and bush bucks, and domestic animals from cattle to dog; among the invertebrates, only the tsetse fly has so far been known as a host.

B 1.1 Characteristics of Trypanosoma

Depending on their way of replicating in the vector, trypanosomes are subdivided into two categories:

Stercoraria: An amastigote forms in humans, the development of which ends in the straight intestine of the vector, e.g. *Triatoma*. An example is *T. cruzi*. The ingested amastigotes replicate in the midgut of *Triatoma* as epimastigotes which bear a flagellum and are finally excreted in the faeces as mature trypomastigotes.

Salivaria: The trypomastigote stage exists in humans and in the vector, but its development ends in the vector (*Glossina*) in the salivary gland. An example is *T. brucei*. In case of the short route, trypanosomes penetrate from the midgut to the salivary gland. In case of the classical route, the pathogenic agents are transported up to the end of the intestine, penetrate into the ectiperitrophic space and then migrate to the front end of the midgut within 10–20 days, from where they penetrate into the hyopharynx. Then they infect the salivary gland.

Trypomastigotes move in body liquids such as blood. They are approximately 10 µm long, 3 µm wide, and bear of flagellum of 10 µm in length which is attached to the body via a pterygium. Intracellularly, there is a large nucleus, kinetoplast, cytoplasmatic granula and the usual cellular organelles (fig. 4). The kinetoplast is a complex DNA-containing mitochondrion which in the case of *T. brucei* spans the entire body. Only *T. cruzi* replicates in humans intracellularly as amastigote as described for *Leishmania*. *T. brucei* has no intracellular form and circulates in blood and tissue fluids as trypomastigote. Trypanosomes can express various different proteins on the surface so that they can escape the immune system, e.g. after cell passage.

B 1.2 Infection and Infectious Disease

T. cruzi: After rubbing the trypomastigotes which are present in the faeces of the bug into the skin, the pathogen replicates and spreads within the body. A chagom forms locally, consisting of oedema and inflammatory cell infiltration. These clinical signs, together with the not very painful swelling of periorbita and lid are called Romaña's sign. The local muscular and tissue cells contain trypomastigotes and amastigotes. The infected cell is lysed, and trypanosomes are released.

Pseudocysts may form in the tissue, which are filled with amastigotes. Very frequently, there is a lymphocytary infiltration. If the cardiac muscle is infected, this will cause necroses which may cause acute cardiac death or chronic cardiac muscle disease, depending on the severity. Another complication arises if the cardiac conduction system and the associated ganglia in the plexus are affected.

Around 10–30% of all infected individuals develop Chagas disease which takes a chronic course. In such cases, the cardiac muscle is the organ most affected. Sudden cardiac death in young adults can be due to the infection of the cardiac muscle and lysis of the muscle cells by *T. cruzi*. Arrhythmia occurs frequently in infected individuals. Other symptoms include megacolon, megaoesophagus, the lumen of which can be dilated by over 10 cm due to paralysis of the nerves of the plexus myentericus. The tissue affected shows strong lymphocytary infiltration.

General signs of the infection include fever and exhaustion, anorexia, lymphoid adenopathy, and minor hepatosplenomegaly. Meningoencephalitis seldom occurs. The intermediary phase, in which high antibody titres against *T. cruzi* are present, follows the acute disease. After several years or decades, the chronic symptomatic Chagas disease follows, affecting the inner organs and showing cardiac arrhythmia and thromboembolism with possible death within several months or years. Even if the course is asymptomatic, immune suppression leads to reactivation of trypanosome replication with general infection of the organs and finally death.

T. brucei: Around 300 trypanosomes form a human infectious dose [56]. After a sting by the tsetse fly, replication occurs in the local tissue which is then invaded by inflammatory cells. The local lymph nodes swell up and finally become fibrotic. These symptoms are followed by hepatosplenomegaly, infection of the cardiac muscle, kidneys, bone marrow and also the skin. Anaemia occurs through accelerated lysis of the red blood cells, which increases by the burden of trypanosome components. Bleeding occurs in the event of thrombocytopenia. A typical sign is when the central nervous system is affected, initially starting in the arachnoidal cavity and the ventricles, then in the entire cavity containing the liquor cerebrospinalis. The latter is rich in protein and contains cells including mononuclear cells such as the special morula cells (also called Marshalko cells).

The incubation period is 5 days to 3 weeks until a local inflammation site is formed. For *T. brucei gambiense*, 1–2 years elapse

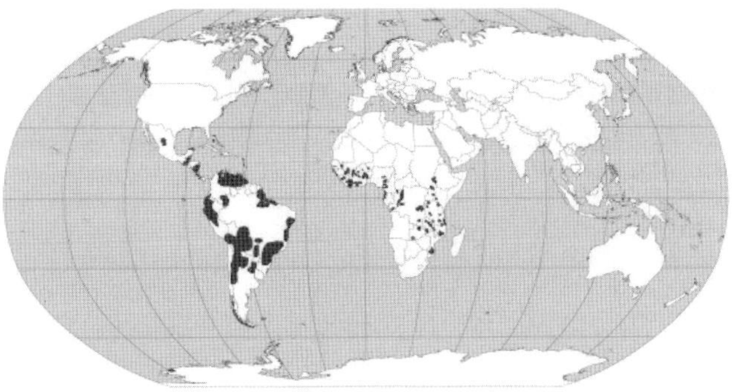

Fig. 5. Distribution of *T. cruzi* in South America and *T. brucei* in Africa, derived from the information generally accessible in 2008.

until the brain is affected; for *T. brucei rhodesiense*, this period is 3–6 months. The disease may subside spontaneously.
General signs, as described above, include fever, lymphadenopathy, oedema, myocarditis, and neuralgia. The disease with increasing apathy and wasting away of the personality, ends in sleeping sickness with chronic meningoencephalitis, if left untreated. Initially, only a deterioration of the mental state is present, followed by mania, hemiplegia, and finally death.

B 1.3 Epidemiology

T. cruzi: The transmitting agents are blood-sucking kissing bugs which replicate in the gaps of brick work, particularly clay tiles or fissures in the tree bark of particularly rural areas. Many wild animals act as hosts. In the latter, as well as in humans, trypanosomes replicate intracellularly as amastigotes, are ingested by the bugs with the blood meal, mature in the rectum (epimastigotes) and are excreted with the faeces during the blood meal (trypomastigotes). They usually enter the body via small skin lesions, conjunctivae, or mucosae during smearing of the bug faeces, which causes a strong itching irritation. Many cells of the body are infected in which amastigotes form afresh. Humans are non-essential hosts in the infection cycle.
In line with the wild animal reservoir and the habitat for the development of *Triatoma*, *T. cruzi* has a cluster-shaped geographical distribution between the south of the USA and Argentina (fig. 5). More than 150 animal species have been described, in which *T. cruzi* replicates. They partly become infected when eating kissing bugs, e.g. armadillo.
Vectors for the transmission of *T. cruzi* to humans include *Triatoma infestans* (fig. 6), and *Rhodnius prolixius*, to a lesser extent *Panstrongylus megistus*, which are wide-spread in rural areas, and, above all, sting at night. Therefore, children living under primitive hygienic conditions, stung in their sleep, are affected particularly frequently (cf. Romaña's sign as described in section B 1.2).
The prevalence of the *T. cruzi* infection in the poor rural population of South America can exceed 9%. Roughly 12% of the infected individuals die of Chagas disease, corresponding to about 45,000 individuals in the two Americas yearly. Combatting *Triatoma* is simple theoretically, but it fails due to economic and political obstacles and the lack of consistent preventive action.
Tourists returning from Latin America to Europe can be *T. cruzi*-infected [57], and *Trypanosoma* can be transmitted by blood donation (cf. sections B 2.1 and B 2.2).
T. brucei: The affected region in Africa is between the northern and southern 20th parallel, ranging more or less from Senegal/Gambia in the west to Botswana/Zimbabwe in the south (fig. 5). Transmission depends on the occurrence of the tsetse fly (*Glossina morsitans*, *G. swynnertoni*, *G. palipides*), which prefers low shrubbery near large animal herds, sucks the blood of the animals and lays its eggs in the faeces of the animals.
Depending on the effectiveness of programmes of combating the tsetse fly, the geographical distribution of sleeping sickness and its incidence vary. A high probability of *T. brucei* transmission persists in the African wild animal reservations [58]. Domestic animals, particularly pigs, act as a reservoir for *T. brucei*, but also antilopes, bushbucks, and Cape buffalos. Some *Glossina* species, e.g. *G. palipides*, are adapted to the human habitat, thus contributing to the regionally increased occurrence of *T. brucei* [59].

B 1.4 Detection Methods and Their Significance

A *T. cruzi/brucei* infection can occur if a donor/recipient has spent a longer period of time in a region with a high degree of infection or spent some time in the region as tourist under primitive conditions of hygiene. Infection with trypanosomes occurred e.g. by a sting from *Triatoma* or *Glossinia* or if he/she received a blood transfusion in an endemic region.

B 1.4.1 Serological Detection (Antibody and Antigen Tests, So-Called Immunological Tests)

T. cruzi: For this chronic infection, the detection of IgM against *Trypanosoma* is of little informational value. Many ELISAs with differing antigen preparations for the detection of IgG are currently commercially available [60, 61], which are also used for the testing of blood donors. The line immunoassay can be used as confirmation test [60]. Many of the tests show low sensitivity and specificity, and display cross-reactions with *Leishmaina*, *Plasmodium* and other protozoae as well as with *Treponema palladium*. In endemic regions, partly 2 or 3 ELISAs are used for the screening of blood donations because of the low specificity.
In Brazil new (rapid) tests for the detection of the *T. cruzi* antibodies on the basis of immunochromatography reach a specificity of 99% at a sensitivity of approximately 93% [62].
T. brucei: To determine exposure, a card agglutination test (CATT) has been developed which is positive 3–4 weeks post infection and reaches a sensitivity of roughly 70–80% [59]. In addition, a latex agglutination test is available displaying a specificity of 96–99% at a sensitivity of 70–100% [63].

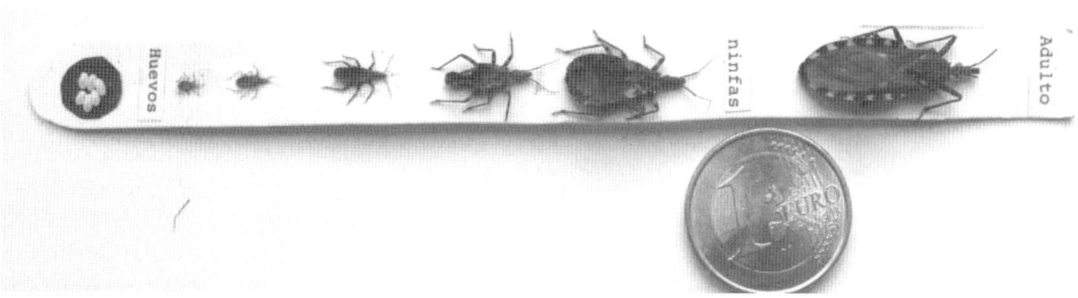

Fig. 6. Kissing bug of the triatoma genus, which is a vector for the transmission of *T. cruzi*. The figure shows the eggs (left), then the nymph stages, and the adult bug (right). The figure also shows sizes of the bugs as compared with a 1-Euro coin. The preparation originates from the Instituto de Investigaciones en Ciencias de la Salud, Asuncion, Paraguay.

Antigen tests for *Trypanosoma* surface proteins based on ELISA or agglutination have so far shown insufficient specificity [59].

B 1.4.2 Isolation of the Pathogen

Xenodiagnosis

Traditionally, for enriching the trypanosomes, the mouse is inoculated with the suspected material, usually blood or tissue . High concentrations of trypanosomes can be found in the blood of the animals after few weeks, and can be detected microscopically after Giemsa staining (fig. 4). Feeding infected material to *Triatoma* is another method used in some specialised laboratories in South America.

Cell Culture

Cell culture systems have been used, usually by employing a feeder layer that can be formed by more than 20 different cell lines, but have been of no significance for the diagnostics of *T. brucei* [64]. L929 cells are suitable for culturing *T. cruzi* [65]. *T. cruzi* can be cultured both in cell-free, and in cell-containing medium [66]. First culturing attempts date back to 1904, the so-called tomato medium [67]; this shows that trypanosomes are relatively undemanding as regards the conditions under which they replicate.

B 1.4.3 Detection by Microscope

The quantity of trypanosomes in peripheral blood is partly very low during chronic infection. Therefore, detection by microscope displays low sensitivity and plays a moderate role. In the acute phase of the infection, a sufficient amount of trypanosomes can be detected over a few days. Histologically, large quantities of trypomastigotes can be detected following biopsy or post mortem examination in the case of *T. cruzi* and *T. brucei*, and large quantities of amastigotes can be detected in the case of *T. cruzi* above all in the cardiac muscle and the intestine.

B 1.4.4 Genome Detection

T. cruzi: Since some genomic sequences are repetitive in kinetoplasts of trypanosomes [68], with roughly 100,000–120,000 copies per parasite, it is possible to detect 1–2 parasites per reaction assay, normally 100–200 µl, using PCR [69, 70]. The amplificates thus obtained have a size of 200–300 base pairs (bp) [71]. PCR is more sensitive than the methods of xenodiagnosis [72].

PCR tests were also developed to determine the success of treatment with benznidazol [73] or nifurtimox [74]. An observation period of several months is necessary to recognise a drop in the PCR amplificates on a quantitative basis. During treatment, a selection of resistant strains can occur. Appropriate analyses show that sub-populations of *T. cruzi* are present in roughly 12% of the cases, and provide proof for the major genetic heterogeneity of the circulating trypanosomes [75].

T. brucei: A PCR was described taking into account the heterogeneity of the *Trypanosoma* strains present in Cameroon, and amplifying sectors within the mobile genetic elements [76], furthermore, a real-time PCR in which the 177 bp repeat satellite DNA is detected [77]. The PCR analysis was able to prove that an infection with *T. brucei* was established in the tsetse fly after 11 days. After 29 days, the trypanosomes were mature, and after 47 days, they could be detected in the saliva [78]. PCR can also be used to analyse isometanidium resistance [1]. The significance of positive PCR results which could not be confirmed by other parasitologic detection methods remains unclear due to the variable specificity [63].

B 2 Blood and Plasma Donors

In Germany, blood and plasma donors are not tested for *Trypanosoma*. No publications on transmissions by blood or blood products exist in Germany which would currently justify such tests from an infectiological point of view.

B 2.1 Prevalence and Incidence in Donor Populations

In Los Angeles, were a high portion of individuals intending to donate blood are of Mexican origin (so-called Hispanidos), between 0.001% and 0.002% have been exposed to or infected with *T. cruzi* [79]. Leiby et al. [80] have indicated a higher prevalence of 0.15% in Los Angeles, CA, and 0.09% in Miami, FL. In endemic regions, transmission by blood is not a rare event. The probability is around 0.75% of the donations in Mexico [81]. *Trypanosoma* transmission also occurs in North America if individuals from endemic regions without clinical symptoms

act as donors [82]. *T. cruzi* has also been transmitted by heart and other organ transplantations in the USA [83], and in Europe, namely Spain, by transplantations of bone marrow [84].
In South America, the prevalence of a *T. cruzi* exposure referred to 100 donors, determined by antibody tests, is 4.5 in Argentina, 9.9 in Bolivia, 1.0 in Guatemala, 2.8 in Paraguay and less than 1.0 in the remaining South American countries. *T. cruzi* occurs in all South American countries [85]. In Brazil, about 0.6% of the blood donations are *Trypanosoma* antibody-positive and are rejected. Within Brazil, there are considerable geographical differences concerning prevalence [31]. In Toronto, Canada, 1,317 blood donors had a possible risk of acquiring *T. cruzi* judged on the basis of their travel destinations and their country of birth, but none of them tested antibody-positive [86]. In California, USA, on the other hand, the parasite was detectable by means of PCR in 33 out of 51 *T. cruzi* antibody-positive blood donors (63%) two decades after immigration, and in 3 individuals also by means of culturing [87].

B 2.2 Definition of Exclusion Criteria

The exclusion criteria in compliance with the guidelines of the Bundesärztekammer and the Paul-Ehrlich-Institut apply for the exclusion of potentially infectious donors [29, 30].
Individuals who show symptoms as described in section B 1.2 and have spent a part of their lifetime in an endemic region [cf. 1] shall be excluded from the donation. Among Latin American immigrants in Berlin, 2% of those who fall into this category, were exposed to *T. cruzi* [88]. Only part of these individuals would be excluded from donating blood due to the current exclusion criteria with respect to a possible malaria transmission.
In 2003, in Madrid, 6 of 659 (0.9%) donors born in *T. cruzi*-endemic regions were antibody-positive [31]. In Spain and Italy, donors originating from endemic regions are deferred from donation for 6 months [31].

B 2.3 Donor Testing and Significance

A testing for *Trypanosoma* or antibodies in donors is not performed in Germany and is not indicated based on the epidemiological situation. Most of the serological tests are of little informational value due to low sensitivity and specificity (cf. section B 1.4). The infection could be identified better by means of PCR than by means of serological tests (cf. section B 1.4).

B 2.4 Donor Interviews

Because of a possible transmission of malaria, donors are interviewed regarding a short or long-term stay in tropical and endemic regions. There are no donor interviews regarding stings by kissing bugs or tsetse flies and periods under simple hygienic conditions. If endemic regions overlap with those where malaria is transmitted, the donor is deferred for 6 months.

B 2.5 Donor Information and Counselling

Information can be provided in connection with travelling to tropical regions. No information is given regarding *Trypanosoma*, the possible risk of *Trypanosoma* transmission and advice concerning the acute clinical symptoms and the chronic course of the infection.
The infection with *Trypanosoma* is not notifiable. Therefore, reliable infection epidemiology data are not available.

B 3 Recipient

B 3.1 Prevalence and Incidence of Blood-Associated Infections and Infectious Diseases in Recipient Populations

No data have been collected on the prevalence and incidence of *Trypanosoma* infections in blood recipients in Germany. In the past 20 years, no reports have been compiled on an infection of *Trypanosoma* transmitted within Germany or on suspected transmission by blood; the same applies to other European countries such as Spain, Italy and France [31].

B 3.2 Immune Status (Resistance, Existing Immunity, Immune Response, Age, Exogenous Factors)

Even if an individual's immune reaction is unimpaired, he or she can be infected with *T. cruzi* if the latter have been rubbed into the skin from the faeces of the arthropode. The infection has a chronic course with clinical manifestation only in 10–30% of the infected individuals (cf. section B 1.2). As immunity decreases, *Trypanosoma* can spread in the body again [74, 82]. In case of *T. brucei*, a sting by the tsetse fly which is painful and therefore clearly perceivable must have preceded.

B 3.3 Severity and Course of the Disease

The infection can be of lethal outcome in case of clinical manifestation and without treatment, partly also under treatment, showing acute heart failure, complications of megaoesophagus and megacolon as well as cerebral defects (cf. section B 1.2).

B 3.4 Therapy and Prophylaxis

T. cruzi: Successes of treatment of Chagas disease are still not satisfactory. Nifurtimox, a nitrofuran derivative, was manufactured by Bayer (Lampit®, Leverkusen, Germany; 8–10 mg/kg body weight for 60–90 days) and used for 20 years. It reduces the symptoms and the death rate, but has considerable adverse effects in around 70% of the patients. Benznidazole (Rochagan® or Radanil® Roche, Basel, Switzerland; 5 mg/kg body weight for 60 days) is of similar effectivity and has adverse effects similar to those of Nifurtimox. For this reason, only patients showing symptoms receive treatment, and a cure is only achieved in 10% of the cases.

Posaconazol (Noxafil®, Essex Pharma, Munich, Germany) can be efficacious according to the first few studies, whereas fluconazol, ketoconazol, veronazol and itraconazol show no effect. IFN-γ, if administered in the acute phase, can eliminate the protozoae [55]. Possible approaches to treatment derive from the interference of peptides with the dimer formation of enzymes as shown on pathogen-specific triosephosphate-isomerase [89].

T. brucei: Suramin was introduced by Bayer as the first medicinal product about 100 years ago. It shows considerable adverse effects. Pentamidine, administered i.m. is of considerably better efficacy and is used today. A cure can only partly be achieved. Dihydroxyacetone in low doses leads to killing of *T. brucei* in cell culture and is possibly suitable for treatment [90]. Difluoromethylornithin and melarsoprol can be used for the treatment of *T. brucei gambiense* infection in Africa with a success rate of around 80% [91]. In this study, antibodies against *T. brucei gambiense* are measured using a latex test.

No chemotherapy and no vaccine are available for the prevention of *Trypanosoma* transmission. Vaccine candidates that have been tested so far have not shown sufficient potency.

B 3.5 Transmissibility

Around 65 laboratory transmissions of *T. cruzi* are known, out of which 11 were caused by parenteral lesions, 3 by contact with the mucosae and 2 by a vector sting [42]. Only 1 of the 6 reported laboratory transmissions with *T. brucei* did not occur in Europe, 5 of the transmissions occurred by sting lesions [42]. Laboratory transmissions of *T. brucei* should occur more frequently in endemic regions of Africa; however, they are not documented.

In a WHO study, estimates of transmissions of *T. cruzi* by blood transfusions in South America for 2000/2001 show the following figures for transmissions per 1,000 donations: 68 for Bolivia, 11 for Chile, 2 for Columbia, 29 for Costa Rica, 11 for Guatemala, 360 for Mexico, 2 for Nicaragua, 52 for Panama and 1 for Paraguay [85]. It can be assumed that these figures are at the lower end of the scale for transmissions which occurred. In blood and cellular blood products, *Trypanosoma* also remains infectious if cooled down to 4 °C. It can be assumed that plasma products do not contain infectious trypanosomes because of their manufacturing procedure.

B 3.6 Frequency of Administration, Type and Amount of Blood Products

Low contamination of a blood component can be sufficient to transmit *Trypanosoma* infection. It can be assumed that transmission in Germany does not take place, or at least extremely rarely, since no transmissions of *Trypanosoma* by blood transfusion or blood products have been reported so far.

B 4 Blood Products

B 4.1 Infectious Load of the Starting Material and Test Methods

It can be assumed that the burden in the starting material is very low in Germany. Test methods for the antibodies formed against *Trypanosoma* are available. However, they are of little use due to low specificity and prevalence. Since no cases of *Trypanosoma* transmission have been reported, it is currently not necessary to introduce the tests.

B 4.2 Methods for Removal and Inactivation of the Infectious Agent

In cellular blood products, high parasitaemia is present only in the acute phase of the infection. Trypanosomes can be accumulated in macrophages. In the case of leucocyte depletion of blood, a marked reduction of the pathogenic agents takes place by removal of the *Trypanosoma*-bearing cells and, in addition, by adhesion of the trypanosomes to the matrix of the filter material based on the negative surface charge [45].

When using sterile filtered plasma, *Trypanosoma* has no significance since the pathogen is retained in the filter [45]. In fractionation of plasma for the preparation of products such as coagulation factors and immunoglobulin, trypanosomes are inactivated and/or removed by sterile filtration.

Inactivation in cell-containing products: Up to 5 $\log_{10}$ trypanosomes can be killed by means of amotosalen and UV irradiation, if grown in cell culture and added to the buffy coat, independently of the *T. cruzi* strain used [92].

B 4.3 Feasibility and Validation of Procedures for Removal/ Inactivation of the Infectious Agent

Blood and/or blood products can be experimentally contaminated with *T. cruzi*, and their depletion and/or inactivation can be evaluated. Because of the extremely low prevalence of *Trypanosoma* infections in Germany, this examination of the depletion is currently not indicated, but could be performed since the technical preconditions are present [92]. Handling *Trypanosoma* requires a safety level 2 laboratory.

Trypanosoma can cause chronic infection in 10–30% of the individuals which can be fatal after illness for months or years. *T. cruzi* and *T. brucei* transmissions depend on the presence of vectors (*Triatoma* and *Rhodnius* or *Glossina*) which do not occur in Central Europe.

Till to date, no *Trypanosoma* transmissions via blood, bone marrow or organ donation have been reported in Germany. After assessment the existing epidemiological and pathogenetic data for transmission and manifestation of *Trypanosoma*, the following preventive steps are currently considered as indicated:

- Exclusion of all donors who received a blood transfusion in the endemic regions of Central and South America and Africa.
- Temporary exclusion of donors after a stay in *Trypanosoma*-endemic regions for 6 months. The *Trypanosoma*-infected regions partly overlap with the malaria endemic regions (fig. 5).
- Exclusion of donors whose centre of activity was temporarily in *Trypanosoma*-endemic regions for 6 months following the time of leaving the endemic region and admission to blood donation only after a decision by a doctor.

C *Babesia* spp.

The pathogenic agent was identified by Victor Babes in the red blood cells of cattle suffering from febrile haemoglobinuria in Romania in 1888. In 1893, a similar agent, described as *Pyrosoma*, was described in Texas. This pathogen today bears the name *Babesia bigemina* [93]. In 1957, *Babesia divergens* was described post mortem in a farmer from Yugoslavia who had undergone splenectomy. In 1969, in Massachusetts *Babesia microti* was found in a man suffering from fever and headache [93].

C 1 Current Knowledge about the Pathogen

Babesia is a member of the Apicomplexa family (apical microtubule complex), in the order of Piroplasmidora and the Theileriidae family, together with *Plasmodium* and *Toxoplasma* as well as other protozoae such as *Cryptosporidium*, *Isospora*, *Microsporidia*, and *Sarcocystis*. Babesias are essentially transmitted by the bite of the tick *Ixodes ricinus* in the Old World, and *Ixodes scapularis* (also called *Ixodes dammini*) in the New World. Babesiosis is a typical zoonosis.

Babesias are either oval or round, of crescent-like shape such as *Plasmodium falciparum*. However, they are smaller and grow within erythrocytes usually as 3–5 trophozoites, which replicate asexually, a process which is known as merogony. Sexual replication only takes place in the tick. This finally leads to formation of sporozoites which invade the salivary gland of the tick.

C 1.1 Characteristics of Babesia

Depending on size, babesias are subdivided into two categories:

- The small variant has a diameter of 1–2.5 µm and includes *Babesia gibsoni* (*canines piroplasma*), *B. microti*, and *Babesia rodhaini*. Trophozoites divide into 4 daughter cells and partly form structures resembling a maltese cross in the Giemsa-stained smear of red blood cells. They can be transmitted in the tick transovarially.
- The large variant has a diameter of 2.5–5 µm and includes *B. divergens*, *Babesia bovis*, *Babesia canis*, and *Babesia odocoilei*. Trophozoites of this type divide into two daughter cells. They are transmitted in the tick non-transoviarially.

The nuclear *small* subunit ribosomal DNA (nss-rDNA) is used for the further characterisation of babesias. From the point of view of genetic code analysis, *B. divergens* is a member of the small type, but as far as its morphology is concerned, it forms part of the large type. Small babesias are more similar to *Theileria* than to large babesias. Babesias are not host-specific. They infect various animals, including humans. *B. divergens* causes babesiosis in Europe, *B. microti* in North America, above all at the East Coast and in the Great Lake region. Not all known *Babesia* strains have so far been classified, and not all *Babesia* strains can infect all animal species.

C 1.1.1 Replication in the Tick

Around 10 h after the blood meal, *Babesia*-infected red cells aggregate in the gut of the tick, and the cytosome, an endocytic organelle, is formed. Around 40–50 h later, the microtubules condense at one end and form the so-called 'ray body'. That way, the basis is formed for fusion of the gametes into the zygote. The zygote penetrates into the gut cell of the tick, then enters the haemolymph and develops into ookinetes which migrate into the salivary gland. There, the sporoblast is formed which replicates by sporogony (sporozoites) at warm temperatures. Sporogony can also happen during the sucking action on the infested animal, through the warming up process. One sporoblast can produce up to 10,000 sporozoites.

C 1.1.2 Replication in Vertebrates

Around 10,000 sporozoites are deposited in the victim's skin, and from there, they probably directly invade red blood cells and develop to merozoites. Merozoite release leads to lysis of the red blood cells. After invading the red blood cells, the merozoites partly changes into trophozoites which can move freely in the cytosol of the cell. The exact mechanism of leaving the cell, also called 'budding' is not known.

C 1.2 Infection and Infectious Disease

Clinical symptoms develop 1–4 weeks after tick bite with malaise, fatigue, lack of appetite and finally fever and chills. The

fever can continue to rise up to 40 °C and persist for months if the patient is immunocompromised. Further symptoms may include photophobia and vomiting. In exceptional cases, exanthema can be found, petechiae are rare. While no lymph node swelling occurs, splenomegaly and hepatomegaly can form.
Laboratory results point to haemolytic anaemia at reduced haptoglobin and increased reticulocyte values. 1–10% of the red blood cells contain babesias if the patient's immune response is intact. In case of immune deficiency, this figure is 85%. Trombocytopenia occurs frequently [93]. In over 25% of immunocompetent individuals, an infection with *B. divergens* can be expected to subside spontaneously without occurrence of clinical symptoms.
In case of Amercian babesiosis, 25% of the infected individuals are hospitalised, around 25% of the hospitalised individuals require treatment in the intensive ward, and 6.5% of these patients die. Causes of death include severe breathing impairment, intravasal coagulation and heart failure. Severe infections can be found at an increased age and in case of immune deficiency [94]. The function of T helper cells plays an important part for overcoming the infection. Removal of the babesias from the tissue and tissue fluid is regulated via the unrestricted function of the macrophages.

C 1.3 Epidemiology

The probability of transmission to humans depends on the prevalence of infected animals in the animal stock. In Southern Switzerland (Tessin), *B. bigemia* was once detected in approximately 1,900 ticks in cows, sheep, red deer and roe in 2004, which was not previously found in that region [95]. In addition to *I. ricinus*, other tick species were examined, and in 6 animals *B. divergens*, in 2 *B. major,* and in 14 *Babesia* were found which were not further characterised [95].
Most of the *Babesia* infection in humans in Europe caused by *B. divergens* were reported from France and England [96]. In 2000, more than 31 cases were reported of which 26 patients (84%) had undergone splenectomy. *B. divergens* was the causative agent in 23 of the infected individuals [97]. One *Babesia* case in a patient who had received splenectomy occurred on the Canary Isles [98]. The first case of *B. divergens/odocoilei* infection in a human was reported from the Hegau region (Germany) in 2007 in a patient who had undergone splenectomy under immunosuppressive treatment. The patient did not remember a tick bite and had never stayed outside Germany [99]. Results of another study showed that in 31 of 3,113 (1%) of the ticks collected in South West Germany, *B. divergens* could be detected by means of PCR [100]. Dogs are another reservoir for *Babesia*. Thus lowland forest ticks (*Dermatocentor reticulatus*) can transmit Babesia to dogs [101, 102]. The significance of lowland forest ticks for the spread of babesias needs to be evaluated in further studies.

In North America most of the human cases of babesiosis are caused by *B. microti*. The number of the cases described exceeds 300 [97]. One case in Germany [103] and one case in Switzerland [104] showed serological reactions against *B. microti*. Infections with *B. canis* and *B. bigemina* in humans were reported from Mexico, other endemic infectious areas are found in West Africa, South Africa, Egypt and China [105].

C 1.4 Detection Methods and Their Significance

The classical method of detection for *Babesia* is the examination of blood smears under the microscope after staining with Giemsa solution or similar methods. At an intraerythrocytic level, 3–5 oval ring shapes can be found, which resemble those of *P. falciparum*, but do not show any other staining besides the blue colour. Extracellular merozoites can be found in severe infections. The so-called maltese cross formation in case of *B. microti* infection is extremely rare.

C 1.4.1 Serological Detection (Antigen and Antibody Tests)
Indirect immunofluorescence is considered as positive if titres >1:64 are reached in case of *B. microti* infection. Titres are usually >1:1,024. Sensitivity depends on the *Babesia* strain used in the immunofluorescence test.
ELISAs based on synthetic peptides of *B. microti* have been developed and are more sensitive than indirect immunofluorescenc [93, 105]. IgG antibodies are usually detectable 2–4 weeks after the occurrence of clinical symptoms. Antigen tests are not commercially available.

C 1.4.2 Culturing
Babesias can be replicated and identified in experimental animals such as hamsters and mice by inoculation of blood of the infected animals [106]. In red blood cells, *B. divergens* can be cultured using the continuous culturing method with high parasite density [96, 107]. Cultured *Babesia* strains adapt to the culture used and lose their virulence.

C 1.4.3 Genome Detection – NAT
By means of PCR, parasitaemia in untreated patients can be detected even 27 months following infection [108, 109]. From that point of view, PCR is the most sensitive method currently available. The target sequence used for the primers is nss-rDNA (nuclear small subunit ribosomal DNA; cf. section C 1.1). Sensitivity is low if primers for *B. microti* are used for the detection of *B. divergens*. The starting material for the PCR is EDTA blood. If *Babesia* DNA is detected in patient blood, this is an indicator for an active infection. If the infection is treated successfully, *Babesia* DNA is no longer detectable in the blood few days later [109, 110]. Detection of *Babesia* (in-situ PCR) using PCR is possible on blood smears [111].

C 2 Blood and Plasma Donors

C 2.1 Prevalence and Incidence in Donor Populations

Only one publication exists on analysing a blood donor collective for the occurrence of *Babesia* in Germany. Among 120 healthy blood donors, indirect immunofluorescence revealed 1.7% (2 of 120) individuals with antibodies [103] (cf. section C 3.1 for specificity). Two of 298 foresters in Southern Germany who, for professional reasons, had a higher risk of exposure to ticks showed antibodies reacting with *B. microti*, but were free of parasitaemia [112]. Two of 190 blood donors in France revealed antibodies against *B. divergens* [96].
Three (0.4%) of 848 blood donors in Connecticut who had reported a tick bite, and 6 (0.6%) of the 1,007 non-interviewed donors used as controls had antibodies against *Babesia* [113]. When the examination was repeated in 2005, 24 (1.4%) from the endemic region and 6 (0.3%) from the non-endemic region out of 1,745 donors altogether had *Babesia* antibodies. In 19 seropositive donors, *Babesia* DNA could be detected in 10 (53%) donors using PCR. The peak of *Babesia* incidence in the USA was reached in July [114]. In the USA, it is assumed that around 50 *Babesia* transmissions occurred by blood transfusions [31].

C 2.2 Definition of Exclusion Criteria

The general guidelines of the Bundesärztekammer and the Paul-Ehrlich-Institut [29, 30] apply to the exclusion of potentially infectious donors. General exclusion criteria that may point to a *Babesia* infection include fever, headache, fatigue and exhaustion, more rarely arthralgia. Anaemia is a typical symptom of chronic *Babesia* infection.
The question for tick bite in the past is a very inaccurate parameter for the prevention of *Babesia* infection [114]. Blood donors remembering tick bite are deferred from donation for 4 weeks, as a preventative measure, also to prevent other viral and bacterial infections.

C 2.3 Donor Testing and Significance

Testing of blood donors for *Babesia* antibodies is not performed in Germany. Based on the low prevalence of *Babesia* infections and the absence of reports on the transmission of *Babesia* spp. by blood transfusion in Germany, such tests are currently not necessary as long as the epidemiological situation does not change (cf. section C 1.3).
A great number of *Babesia* transmissions occurred in the USA from asymptomatic donors even if the blood was kept refrigerated for 5–35 days and even if the blood was frozen in the presence of glycerol [115–119]. The first transfusion-associated case of babeosis was reported in Canada in 2001 [120]. *Babesia* can be transmitted by an asymptomatic donor over a period of 6 months [121].

C 2.4 Donor Interviews

In compliance with the guidelines, donor interviews on the general symptoms of *Babesia* infection (cf. section C 2.2) are not carried out. Questions are asked referring to a tick bite depending on the season. No interviewing takes place concerning *Babesia* infection since the clinical symptoms in connection with this infection are not known among the general population; based on the epidemiological situation, interviewing would be of little informational value and barely successful. Since no case of *Babesia* infection caused by blood transfusion has so far been reported in Germany, a special interview is not required.

C 2.5 Donor Information and Counselling

Since *Babesia* infections and the clinical symptoms of *Babesia* are very rare, it is currently not necessary to provide advice in the blood donation centres.

C 3 Recipients

The incubation period of *B. microti* infections via blood is between 17 days and 9 weeks, for infections transmitted by ticks it is 1–4 weeks [119, 122].

C 3.1 Prevalence and Incidence of Blood-Associated Infections and Infectious Diseases in Recipient Populations

Prevalence and incidence depend on the endemic region, essentially are the rate of infection in the animal reservoir (cf. section C 1.3), tick density, season, and the corresponding tick activity and leisure activities of the recipients.
A study is available concerning this topic [103]. In the Rhine-Main region, 11.5% (26 of 225) of the individuals exposed to tick bite were *Babesia* antibody-positive (indirect immunofluorescence, no confirmation test) as opposed to 2% (2 of 120) of blood donors. In the collective examined which included, 467 sera, reactivity against *Babesia* was higher against *B. microti* with 5.4% (25 of 467) than against *B. divergens* with 3.6% (17 of 467). The cut-off of the antibody dilution was 1:64 for *B. microti* and 1:128 for *B. divergens* (cf. section C 1.4).
In the USA, one case of *Babesia* transmission by heart transplantation [123] and three cases by kidney transplantation were reported [124–126].

C 3.2 Immune Status (Resistance, Existing Immunity, Immune Response, Age, Exogenous Factors)

Immune deficiency caused by splenectomy promotes *Babesia* replication and leads to severe, often deadly courses of the disease. The immune deficiency, which is also age-related, favours an infection with clinical symptoms [93, 124]. The relatively high prevalence of antibody-positive individuals points to the fact that persons with an unimpaired immune system overcome infection without any signs of disease pointing to babesiosis.

C 3.3 Severity and Course of the Disease

Effective treatment can prevent deaths even in immunosuppressed individuals and patients after splenectomy [119]. The infection with *B. microti* in North America often presents with minor symptoms, such as fatigue or exhaustion, possibly also anaemia (cf. section C 1.2 and C 2.2), or occurs subclinically [93].

C 3.4 Therapy and Prophylaxis

Around 75% of immunocompetent patients infected with *Babesia* have minor clinical signs or overcome the infection with minor clinical symptoms without treatment.
B. microti: Patients after splenectomy and with immune deficiency are treated with clindamycin and oral quinine for 7–10 days. Chloroquine, which is administered for *P. falciparum*, is ineffective. The same applies to medicinal products such as primaquine, pyrimethamine, tetracycline, pentamidine and others. Atovaquone combined with azithromycine leads to death of *Babesia* and shows fewer adverse effects than the combination of clindamycin and quinine. Atovaquone as monotherapy leads to rapid development of resistance [93].
B. divergens: In addition to the combination of clindamycin and quinine, the combination of pentamidine and trimethoprim/sulfamethoxazol can be used. Blood transfusions are indicated for patients with high parasitaemia and strong haemolysis. [93].
Vaccination: No vaccination is currently available against *Babesia*. Attempts at vaccinating against *B. divergens* and *B. bigemia*, including vaccinations in cattle with attenuated babesias, were unsuccessful [127]. Among the recombinant antigens, the RAP-1 protein (rhoptry-associated protein) induced a high antibody and good T-lymphocyte response, but did not confer protective immunity [128]. In vaccinated cattle, immunity is rapidly compromised by *Babesia*, which have an altered amino acid composition in the hypervariable region of the MSA-2 (merozoite surface antigen) [129] or MSA-1, if the latter is used in the vaccination [130].

C 3.5 Transmissibility

Babesia in blood is neither destroyed by cooling down to 4 °C nor by freezing. Consequently, parasite-containing blood is always infectious. *Babesia* was seldom transmitted via blood after kidney or heart transplantations. The infection probably manifested itself due to immune suppression [123]. In 1993 in Connecitcut, the risk of *Babesia* transmission by red blood cells was higher than that of *Borrelia* transmission with 0.17%. *Borrelia* could not be detected in any of the blood samples. In the cited study, no pathogenic agent was transmitted via platelets [131].
Till to date, no accidental transmissions of *Babesia* during laboratory work have been reported [42].

C 3.6 Frequency of Administration, Type and Amount of Blood Products

With increased administration of red blood cells, the theoretical risk of *Babesia* transmission rises also. Since no transmissions have been reported in Germany so far, the risk of increased application is also negligible. To obtain more accurate data, epidemiologically verified results should be awaited from studies with validated tests.

C 4 Blood Products

C 4.1 Infectious Load of the Starting Material and Test Methods

Apart from the study by Hunfeld et al. [103] on blood donors, no detailed studies have been conducted on the burden in blood donations in Germany. As described in section C 1.4, *Babesia* can be detected by microscopy in case of higher infections in red blood cells. However, nucleic acid detection by PCR [108–110] is a better and more sensitive method (cf. section C 1.4).
Since *Babesia* is present in the blood in cell-bound form, the burden in the plasma has no significance.

C 4.2 Methods for Removal and Inactivation of the Infectious Agent

Since *Babesia* growth is preferably intraerythrocytic, the protozoon cannot be removed from cellular blood components by methods such as filtration. Since up to 10% of the cell fraction of granulocyte concentrates consist of red blood cells and also platelet concentrates contain erythrocytes, *Babesia* cannot be removed from these products either.
In blood plasma, *Babesia* is not contained in quantities sufficient to cause infection [121, 123]. Because of their size, free

babesias can be retained by suitable filters (0.22 μm) [64, 119]. Therefore, *Babesia* has no significance for the use of sterile filtered plasma. Babesias are depleted and/or inactivated during fractionation of plasma for the production of preparations such as coagulation factors and immunoglobulin.

C 4.2.1 Inactivation

Photoinactivation of *Babesia* in plasma with amotosalen and UV irradiation is possible; more than 5.5 log_{10} could be inactivated following spiking [132].

C 4.3 Feasibility and Validation of Procedures for Removal/ Inactivation of the Infectious Agent

Since *Babesia* can be replicated in culture [64, 133], spiking of blood is theoretically possible. However, since the pathogenic agent's growth is intraerythrocitic, the method for measuring the burden on the red blood cells involves a high workload. In addition, additives such as foetal calf serum impair the growth of *Babesia* in culture [134]. An animal model involving mouse or hamster could be used for validation of the inactivation method, since many *Babesia* strains also grow in these experimental animals [64].

C 5 Assessment

Babesia is a parasite that grows within erythrocytes and is transmissible from animals to humans via ticks. The infection is often resolved spontaneously, but it can also have a subclinical course with persisting parasitaemia for several months. In immunocompromised individuals in North America, e.g. after splenectomy, severe, partly deadly infections were caused by *B. microti*, and in Europe by *B. divergens*, when treatment with combinations of quinine and clindamycin or with atovaquone and azithromycin were not started promptly.

B. divergens and similar species are also present in Germany [99]. Since transfusion-associated *Babesia* transmission have so far not been reported in Germany, the presence of these agents does not justify general testing of all blood donations for markers of a *Babesia* infection. Clinical signs of chronic babesiosis are noticeable with severe anaemia, liver and spleen swelling, high LDH and reduced haptoglobin values as a sign of haemolysis. A *Babesia* infection can be diagnosed microscopically in the blood smear with high parasite density during the acute phase of infection with intraerythrocytary merozoites. Cases of transmission would have been identified using these diagnostic parameters in the past.

Based on the epidemiological situation, the small number of cases, and the missing reports on preventing a potential *Babesia* transmission via blood transfusion, there is currently no action required in Germany that goes beyond the general exclusion criteria.

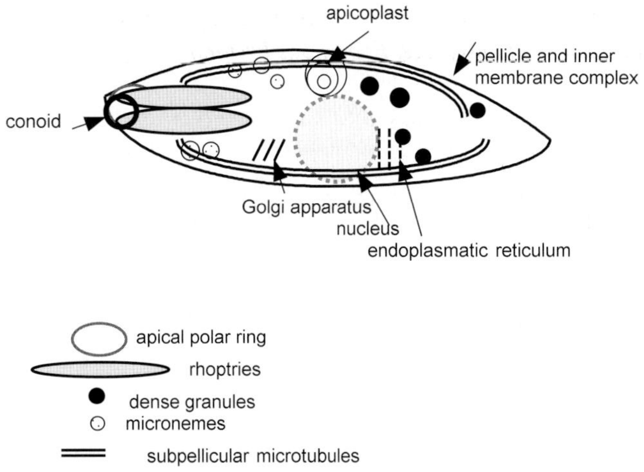

Fig. 7. Schematic presentation of the cell structure of apicomplexa, which include for example Babesia, Plasmodium and Toxoplasma.

D *Toxoplasma gondii*

D 1 Current Knowledge about the Pathogen

Toxoplasma has a world-wide geographical distribution, and more than a quarter of the world population is infected with this agent. Since transmissions from humans to humans by social contacts have so far not been observed, with the exception of pregnancies, the disease is a typical zoonosis. Vertical transmission of the infection from the mother to the foetus with severe malformation is only possible if primary infection occurs during pregnancy.

Toxoplasma was discovered independently in 1908 by Charles Nicolle and Louis H. Manceaux [135], while they were looking for *Leishmania* in a rodent (*Ctenodactylus gundi*) in North Africa, and by Alfonso Splendore in rabbits in Sao Paulo [136]. The first human infection was decribed by Josef Janku in Czechia in 1923 [4], and congenital transmission was discovered by Arne Wolf and David Cowen in the same year and published later [137].

D 1.1 Characteristics of T. gondii

T. gondii are classified as members of *Apicomplexa* (fig. 7) in the class of the *Sporozoae* and occurs in three distinct forms:
- as oocyst which forms sporozoites;
- as tachyzoite, the crescent shaped form which develops when sporozoites infect tissue cells which replicate by longitudinal division in these cells and are then released (particularly affected cells include macrophages, neutrophil granulocytes, ependymal cells and atrocytes), and
- as tissue cyst containing bradyzoites which remain infectious in the cyst for many years.

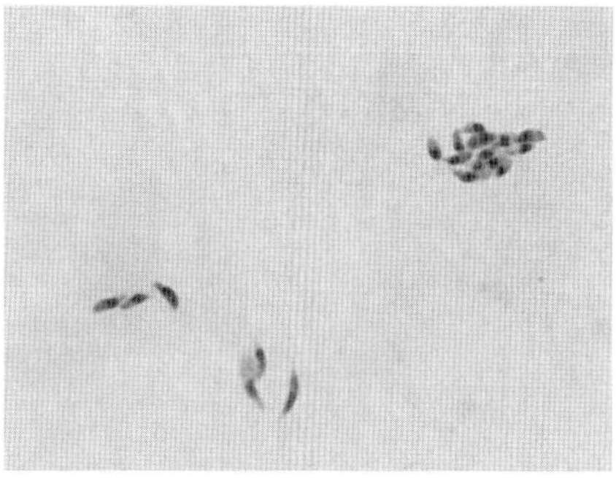

Fig. 8. Crescent shaped toxoplasmas replicated in culture cells. The toxoplasmas have migrated to the supernatant after lysis of the cells. May-Grünwald-Giemsa stain. Preparation from the Friedrich-Löffler-Institut für Medizinische Mikrobiologie (Friedrich-Löffler-Institute for Medical Microbiology), University Hospital, Greifswald, Germany.

Sexual cycles of the development only take place in cats and felides, while asexual replication takes place in many animal species and humans [138].
For *T. gondii*, 3 genotypes can be distinguished: Genotype I and II have been found in congenital toxoplasmosis [139]. Genotype II is the strain most frequently found in humans that has a tendency for reactivation and chronic infection and is also found in 65% of the AIDS patients [140]. Genotype III strains preferentially occur in animals, rarely in humans.
Oocyst: Oocysts are formed in jejunium cells of the intestine of the cat after sporozoites have entered the organism. Sporozoites merge during the sexual cycle after the sporozoites have transformed into gametocytes. Unsporulated oocysts are of 10–12 µm in diameter, they are formed 7–20 days following infection. 10 million oocysts can be excreted per day. Only sporulated oocysts are infectious. They contain 2 sporocysts which in turn contain 4 sporozoites. Sporulation takes 2–3 weeks at a temperature of 11 °C; at 24 °C it takes 2–3 days. Oocysts remain infectious in humid soils for more than 18 months.
Tachyzoite: Tachyzoites have the crescent shaped form with a length of 5–7 µm and a width of 2–3 µm. Tachyzoites can only replicate within cells. The period of division is about 6–8 h. If the number is too high, the cell will burst and the tachyzoites thus released will infect the adjacent cells or cells in other tissues by active propulsion. They are phagocytised by macrophages and are transported by neutrophil granulocytes in blood. A conoid is located at a pole of the tachyzoite which contains 8 organelles (rhoptries and micronemes, fig. 7, 8). The enzymes of the organelles are used to penetrate the cell wall. Tachyzoites are sensitive to desiccation, freezing, thawing, and an acid environment [141].
Bradyzoite: Bradyzoites are located in tissue cysts. They are morphologically distinct from tachyzoites and replicate very slowly. Tachyzoites transform into bradyzoites under the influence of substances such as IFN-γ and heat shock proteins. A tissue cyst can contain more than 1,000 bradyzoites. In the muscle, bradyzoites are inactivated in the tissue system by heating to >67 °C, and by freezing at –20 °C for 24 h. Bradyzoites can migrate from the cyst and transform into tachyzoites [142]. Bradyzoites can remain infectious in tissue for decades [143].

D 1.2 Infection and Infectious Disease

In humans, *Toxoplasma* replicates intracellularly at the entry site without any preference for any cells, no matter whether sporozoites, tachyzoites or bradyzoites are inoculated. Regional lymph nodes act as the primary collection site for released *Toxoplasma*. The clinical outcome in the lymph node is that of histiocytosis accompanied by microabcesses and granuloma with abnormally large Langerhans cells. Tachyzoites can survive in phagocytes if they form parasitophorous vacuoles which protect them from fusion with lysosomes. Even if immunity has been established, intracellular or intra-tissue protozoae cannot be killed. Such cysts can be identified in the brain, eye, cardiac or skeletal muscle of 10% of seropositive individuals [144].
In immunocompetent individuals, infection with *Toxoplasma* leads to chronic or latent infection. Bradyzoites can occasionally be released from tissue cysts [142]. Infection with *Toxoplasma* leads to humoral and cellular immunity which persists life-long by boostering through endogenous or exogenous re-infection. As immunity is established, *Toxoplasma* is eliminated from the blood stream. IFN-γ plays an essential part in immunity establishment [145]. Antibodies of the classes IgG, A, M, and E are formed. Patients with the cell surface marker HLA-DQ3 have a higher probability of developing encephalitis [146].
Typical signs of primary infection only occur in 10–20% of infected individuals. Cervical lymph node swelling is frequently found, which persists and reaches up to 3 cm in size, accompanied by fever, nocturnal sweating, malaise, and muscular pain. Clinical signs resemble those of mononucleosis caused by EBV (Epstein-Barr virus) and CMV (cytomegalovirus). A differential diagnosis should be made to exclude malignant lymphoma such as Morbus Hodgkin. Lymph node swelling can persist several months [138].

D 1.3 Epidemiology

Toxoplasma gondii has a world-wide geographical distribution. Infections in humans are usually caused by eating uncooked or undercooked meat, contaminated vegetables and water, or swallowing oozytes, e.g. in dust. *Toxoplasma* could also be isolated from hen's eggs [147]. Tachyzoites can be transmitted via uncooked goat's milk and can lead to infection [148].
Maternofoetal infections are very rare in Germany (2007: 20 cases reported, 2006: 10 cases, 2005: 18 cases, 2004: 16 cases, 2003: 19 cases, 2002: 17 cases, and 2001: 37 cases; source of data: Robert Koch-Institut). *Toxoplasma* transmissions by blood transfusion and organ transplantations did occur (cf. section D 3.5), furthermore, also those by needle pricks [149].
Arthropods which also feed on faeces (coprophagia), such as cockroaches and flies, albeit rarely, can be transmitters upon entering open wounds or contaminating the mucosae. From that point of view, *Toxoplasma* can also be classified as ranking

among arboprotozoae. *Toxoplasma* antibody incidence in humans increases with age; there is no gender dependency [138]. *Toxoplasma* seroprevalence in Western Europe and Africa (Uganda, Zambia) can amount to up to 50 and 70% respectively [150, 151]. In France, 1,215 (72.2%) of 1,683 HIV-infected individuals were seropositive for *Toxoplasma* [152]. In the USA, the prevalence is lower than in Europe. Among the recruits of the US army, 9.5% were seropositive in 1989, and 14.4% in 1965. 9% of women of child-bearing age in San Francisco, CA, were seropositive in 2003.

D 1.4 Detection Methods and Their Significance

The most suitable method for detecting acute infection in blood or other body fluids is NAT (amplification of *Toxoplasma* DNA). A negative NAT result, however, does not indicate that the material is free from *Toxoplasma* infection since *Toxoplasma* is not equally distributed in blood and tissue. Tachyzoites can be identified in the case of acute infection in histological products, above all lymph nodes. For the detection of chronic infection or exposure, IgG antibody determination is the best suitable methods.

D 1.4.1 Antibody Detection

Antibody tests also detect a high number of exposed individuals among blood donors. These tests are not suitable for distinguishing between infectious and non-infectious donors. The Sabin-Feldman test is rarely used now. The most frequently used test is the ELISA which is not free from false-negative and false-positive results. Immunoblot can be used as a confirmatory test. This test is available from various manufacturers and reaches a sensitivity of 52–67% and a specificity of 96–99% if a postnatal diagnosis is required for congenital infection [153]. In another study, the Western blot reached a sensitivity of 82% and a specificity of 97%. More recent tests show a sensitivity of 99% and specificity of 100% [154]. The differentiation can be made more accurate by means of a two-dimensional immunoblot analysis [155]. The avidity test reveals the duration of an infection only to a limited extent [156].

IgM antibodies decline again after 12–18 months following an immune reaction. IgA antibodies can persist 6–9 months up to 1 year [138, 156]. IgM tests have a low specificity, even if their structure is based on the sandwich principle [157].

It has been reported that IgE antibody determination performs better than IgM determination for differentiating between an acute and a chronic infection [158]. IgE determination can be valuable in detecting acute infection, since IgE antibodies decline after 4–6 months while IgM antibodies only decline after 12–18 months [156].

D 1.4.2 Culturing

Inoculation of the mouse or cell culture are suitable for pathogen isolation. Cell culturing is simpler and faster. Tachyzoites can be detected in the stained sample after only 3–6 days (fig. 7). Peripheral mononuclear cells from the blood of non-*Toxoplasma*-exposed individuals can be used, or granulocytes which would have to be added every 2–3 days. A well-established cell system uses fibroblasts of the MRC5 cell line [159].

D 1.4.3 Antigen Detection

ELISA and agglutination test: An antigen test which probably only recognised tachyzoites was described in 1982 [160], but was not commercialised. Further antigen tests were described in the 1980s and have today been replaced by NAT.

Microscopy: In the microscopic preparation, tachyzoites can be found in the Giemsa stain, if present in large numbers. Fluorescent antibodies have been used to increase sensitivity. However, these antibodies also caused more unspecific staining [161].

D 1.4.4 Genome Detection by Means of NAT

Many methods have been described for *Toxoplasma* DNA PCR, above all for the detection of *Toxoplasma* in AIDS patients [162, 163]. Primers from the B1 gene of *Toxoplasma* are used for amplification. [68]. The gene is present several times (usually 5-fold). More recent methods use real-time PCR [164]. Sensitivity depends on the parasite density in the product. A sensitivity of 64% and a specificity of nearly 100% can be reached using real-time PCR [165].

PCR can be used for genotyping of *Toxoplasma* [166]. Using this method, differentiation takes place by amplification of 5 different genes. When comparing the different PCR methods, real-time PCR is the fastest and FRET (fluorescence resonance energy transfer) or nested PCR is the most sensitive method [167]. PCR is more sensitive for detecting *Toxoplasma* in blood, if leucocytes are used for nucleic acid extraction. One *Toxoplasma* can be detected in enriched leucocytes corresponding to approximately 200 µl blood after a storage period of 1–6 days [168].

D 2 Blood and Plasma Donors

D 2.1 Prevalence and Incidence in Donor Populations

Prevalence depends on the endemic region, the exposure to animals, above all cats, and the age of the individual, and basically corresponds to the prevalence in the general population (cf. section D 1.3). Thus, an antibody prevalence of 0.3–7.6% has been indicated for haematopoietic stem cell donors [169]. Among blood donors in Thailand, a *Toxoplasma* antibody prevalence of 4.9% has been found in 2000 [170]. In the Canton of Zurich, Switzerland, in 1995 a prevalence of 52% and 40% was found among blood donors and women between 20 and 40 years, respectively [171].

D 2.2 Definition of Exclusion Criteria

The general guidelines of the Bundesärztekammer and the Paul-Ehrlich-Institut apply to the exclusion of potentially infectious donors and, in addition, the deferral for 6 months after the symptoms of toxoplasmosis have subsided [29, 30]. Characteristic symptoms of an acute *Toxoplasma* infection include in particular fever, malaise, exhaustion and cervical lymoph node swelling.

D 2.3 Donor Testing and Significance

Testing for *Toxoplasma* or *Toxoplasma* NAT in donors is currently not performed and is not indicated based on the lack of reports on *Toxoplasma* infections in the recipient collective following blood transfusion.

D 2.4 Donor Interviews

Donors are interviewed for signs of inflammation, particularly fever and lymph node swelling after a known *Toxoplasma* infection, however, not for contact with pets or the consumption of insufficiently cooked meat.

D 2.5 Donor Information and Counselling

Since *Toxoplasma* infections and *Toxoplasma*-associated clinical symptoms are very rare in blood donors, it is currently not necessary to provide advice concerning the subject in the blood donation centres. Such advice can be given in any centre of infectious diseases in Germany, if required.

D 3 Recipient

Similarly to donors, the rate of infection among recipients is as high as that of the general population with regional differences and the age-dependent increase in seropositivity. Concerning infections in recipients, differentiation must be made between new infection, re-infection, and reactivation. A distinction is possible only if serological results are available.

D 3.1 Prevalence and Incidence of Blood-Associated Infections and Infectious Diseases in Recipient Populations

The recipient collective in Germany has an antibody prevalence of 20–30%, depending on dietary behaviour and age, and partly also higher with 50 and 70%, as found in Switzerland [171]. Contrary to these findings, the prevalence described in the USA was 9–14% [138] (cf. section D 1.3).

D 3.2 Immune Status (Resistance, Existing Immunity, Immune Response, Age, Exogenous Factors)

The immunological condition is essential for controlling *Toxoplasma* infection. AIDS patients with a CD4 cell number of <200/µl often develop cerebral or pulmonary toxoplasmosis due to endogenous reactivation, which is of fatal outcome when untreated [172].

D 3.3 Severity and Course of the Disease

In case of impaired immune response, including chemotherapy, *Toxoplasma* continues to spread in the body and can lead to acute disease up to 3 years after bone marrow transplantation [159]. *Toxoplasma* can be transmitted via liver transplant and can lead to pneumonia [173]. Pneumonia rarely occurs in immunocompetent individuals [174]. Cerebral toxoplasmosis is of fatal outcome in immunosuppressed patients, if it is not diagnosed early and treated sufficiently [175].
The serious immune suppression after stem cell or bone marrow transplantation may require testing for *Toxoplasma* antibodies in the donor and the recipient [175].

D 3.4 Therapy and Prophylaxis

Drugs used for treatment will inhibit the growth of tachyzoites, but will not damage bradyzoites in the tissue cysts. Pyrimethamine as folic acid antagonist is the most efficacious product. It should be administered in combination with sulfadiazine or clindamycin. Duration of treatment should be at least 3 weeks. On the one hand, azithromycine, clarithromycin, atovaquone, dapsone and trimethoprime-sulfomethroxazol are effective. On the other hand, little experience is available on the duration of treatment using these products [138]. Spiramycine can be administered successfully during pregnancy. In case of severe immune suppression, IFN-γ is administered as a supportive measure in combination with roxithromycine, or pyrimethamine and/or azithromycine.

D 3.5 Transmissibility

Toxoplasma can survive in citrated blood at 4 °C for >50 days [138]. *Toxoplasma* was transmitted by whole blood and by leucocyte concentrates, with leucocytes increasing the risk of transmission [176]. Organ transplantations, too, can cause transmission of *Toxoplasma* [177]. Besides the transmission, reactivation can occur in seropositive transplanted patients. No *Toxoplasma* infection was transmitted through the transfer of haematopoietic stem cells during autologous transplantation (0 of 6,787). However, this did occur during allogenic transplantation in 0.97% of the cases (41 of 4,231) [178]. A pyrimethamine

prophylaxis can probably prevent *Toxoplasma* infection after transplantation with a >80% probability.
47 laboratory infections with *Toxoplasma* have been described, out of which 14 were lesions caused by stinging, 12 without recorded event of an accident, 8 by moistening the mucosa, 8 by oocyst uptake. The mean incubation period was 8.5 days ,with a range of 2 days up to 2 months; most of the patients suffering from the accidents had an incubation period of <13 days [42].

D 3.6 Frequency of Administration, Type and Amount of Blood Products

Non-leucocyte-depleted blood products have an increased risk of causing transmission of *Toxoplasma gondii* tachyzoites. The highest risk is represented by granulocyte concentrates [176]. The more donors are included in the preparation of a granulocyte product, the higher the risk of *Toxoplasma* contamination. Plasma products do not contain any viable tachyzoites since these agents are removed by sterile filtration during the manufacturing process.

D 4 Blood Products

D 4.1 Infectious Load of the Starting Material and Test Methods

Cell-containing blood products can contain *Toxoplasma*. The probability of *Toxoplasma* burden is especially high if a donor is in the acute phase of the infection or in a chronic relapsing phase of the course of infection.

D 4.2 Methods for Removal and Inactivation of the Infectious Agent

Since tachyzoites of *Toxoplasma* mainly occur in phagocytes, the protozoae can be removed effectively (>3 $\log_{10}$) by leucocyte depletion.
Thermoinactivation is effective as from 67 °C [179]. This method cannot be used for cellular blood products and plasma derivatives. The tachyzoites are isolated and inactivated during fractionation and sterilisation of plasma proteins. If sterile filtered fresh frozen plasma is used, *Toxoplasma* has no significance since the pathogenic agent is retained in the filter because of its size [165]. Fresh frozen plasma does not transmit *Toxoplasma* since the agent looses its infectiousness at temperatures of <20 °C. During fractionation of plasma for the manufacture of products such as coagulation factors and immunoglobulin, *Toxoplasma* is depleted and/or inactivated.

D 4.3 Feasibility and Validation of Procedures for Removal/ Inactivation of the Infectious Agent

Since *Toxoplasma* can be replicated in cell culture, spiking of blood and blood products is possible. The essential aspect of *Toxoplasma* contamination, however, is the growth in phagocytes which cannot be simulated by simple spiking, and for which special culturing conditions and spiking with infected leucocytes is required. Adding infected MRC5 cells [159] from cell culture, however, has little similarity to the natural infection process.
If the aim is to test depletion or inactivation in plasma, spiking of plasma with *Toxoplasma* enriched in culture cells can be helpful, analogous with spiking with *Babesia* [132].
Specific methods for elimination or intracellular inactivation have so far not been described.

D 5 Assessment

Toxoplasma gondii has a world-wide geographical distribution, and depending on the human population studied, the infection prevalence can be up to 80%. The progression of the infection is stopped after successful immune response, but can be reactivated in case of immune suppression. Treatment is available only against tachyzoites. The administration of therapeutic drugs cannot inactivate *Toxoplasma* in the dormant state.
No infections by blood transfusions have so far been reported from Germany. Consequently, the donor selection regime and leucocyte depletion appears to prevent such infections. Thus, additional steps, such as the routine testing for *Toxoplasma* antibodies, are not required.

This paper was completed on August 28, 2008, and approved by the German Advisory Committee Blood (Arbeitskreis Blut) on October 29, 2008. It was compiled by the members of the subgroup 'Assessment of Pathogens Transmissible by Blood' of the German Advisory Committee Blood (Arbeitskreis Blut):

Prof. Dr. Lutz Gürtler
Dr. Johannes Blümel
Prof. Dr. Reinhard Burger
Prof. Dr. Christian Drosten
Dr. Albrecht Gröner
Dr. Margarethe Heiden
PD Dr. Martin Hildebrandt
Prof. Dr. Dr. Bernd Jansen
Dr. Thomas Montag-Lessing
Dr. Ruth Offergeld
Prof. Dr. Georg Pauli
Prof. Dr. Rainer Seitz
Dr. Uwe Schlenkrich
Dr. Volkmar Schottstedt
Dr. Johanna Strobel
Dr. Hannelore Willkommen
Prof. Dr. Carl-Heinz Wirsing von König

References

1 Blümel J, Burger R, Drosten C, Gröner A, Gürtler L, Heiden M, Jansen B, Klamm H, Ludwig WD, Montag-Lessing T, Offergeld R, Pauli G, Seitz R, Schlenkrich U, Schottstedt V, Willkommen H, Wirsing von König KH, Knobloch J: Malaria. Transfus Med Hemother 2008;35:122–134.

2 Pozio E: Epidemiology and control prospects of foodborne parasitic zoonoses in the European Union. Parassitologia 2008;50:17–24.

3 Kotton CN: Zoonoses in solid-organ and hematopoietic stem cell transplant recipients. Clin Infect Dis 2007;44:857–866.

4 Cox FE: History of human parasitology. Clin Microbiol Rev 2002;15:595–612.

5 Hoare CA: Early discoveries regarding the parasites of oriental sore. Trans Roy Soc Trop Med Hyg 1938;32:67–92.

6 Jeronimo SM, Sousa ADQ, Pearson RD: Leishmania species: visceral (Kala-Azar), cutaneous, and mucocutaneous leishmaniasis; in Mandell GL, Bennett JE, Dolin R (eds): Principles and Practice of Infectious Diseases, 6th ed. Orlando, Churchill Livingstone, 2005, pp 3145–3156.

7 Burgess NRH, Cowan GO: Medical Entomology. London, Chapman and Hall, 1993.

8 Grogl M, Daugirda JL, Hoover DL, Magill AJ, Berman JD: Survivability and infectivity of viscerotropic *Leishmania tropica* from Operation Desert Storm participants in human blood products maintained under blood bank conditions. Am J Trop Med Hyg 1993;49:308–315.

9 Cardo LJ: Leishmania: risk to the blood supply. Transfusion 2006;46:1641–1645.

10 Moradpour D, Markwalder K, Greminger P, Lüthy R: Visceral leishmaniasis as an opportunistic infection. Case report and literature review. Schweiz Rundsch Med Prax 1990;79:921–926.

11 Martin-Sánchez J, Navarro-Mari JM, Pasquau-Liaño J, Salomón OD, Morillas-Márquez F: Visceral leishmaniasis caused by *Leishmania infantum* in a Spanish patient in Argentina: what is the origin of the infection? Case report. BMC Infect Dis 2004;4:20.

12 Alvar J, Aparicio P, Aseffa A, Den Boer M, Canavate C, Dedet JP, Gradoni L, Ter Horst R, Lopez-Velez R, Moreno J: The relationship between leishmaniasis and AIDS: the second 10 years. Clin Microbiol Rev 2008;21:334–359.

13 Herrmann A, Wohlrab J, Sudeck H, Burchard GD, Marsch WC: Chronic lupoid leishmaniasis. A rare differential diagnosis in Germany for erythematous infiltrative facial plaques. Hautarzt 2007;58:256–260.

14 Weitzel T, Mühlberger N, Jelinek T, Schunk M, Ehrhardt S, Bogdan C, Arasteh K, Schneider T, Kern WV, Fätkenheuer G, Boecken G, Zoller T, Probst M, Peters M, Weinke T, Gförer S, Klinker H, Holthoff-Stich ML; Surveillance Importierter Infektionen in Deutschland (SIMPID) Surveillance Network: Imported leishmaniasis in Germany 2001–2004: data of the SIMPID surveillance network. Eur J Clin Microbiol Infect Dis 2005;24:471–476.

15 Harms G, Schönian G, Feldmeier H: Leishmaniasis in Germany. Emerg Infect Dis 2003;9:872–875.

16 Bogdan C, Schönian G, Bañuls AL, Hide M, Pratlong F, Lorenz E, Röllinghoff M, Mertens R: Visceral leishmaniasis in a German child who had never entered a known endemic area: case report and review of the literature. Clin Infect Dis 2001;32: 302–306.

17 Harms-Zwingenberger G, Bienzle U: Nach Deutschland importierte Leishmaniosen. Dtsch Ärztebl 2007; 104:A3108–3113.

18 Bruckner DA, Labarca JA. Leishmania and Trypanosoma; in Murray PR, Baron EJ, Jorgensen JH, Pfaller MA, Yolken RH (eds): Manual of Clinical Microbiology, 8th ed. Washington, ASM Press, 2003, pp 1960–1969.

19 Lima HC, Bleyenberg JA, Titus RG: A simple method for quantifying Leishmania in tissues of infected animals. Parasitol Today 1997;13:80–82.

20 Le Fichoux Y, Quaranta JF, Aufeuvre JP, Lelievre A, Marty P, Suffia I, Rousseau D, Kubar J. Occurrence of *Leishmania infantum* parasitemia in asymptomatic blood donors living in an area of endemicity in southern France. J Clin Microbiol 1999;6: 1953–1957.

21 Disch J, Caligiorne RB, Maciel F, Oliviera MC, Orsini M, Dias-Neto E, Rabello A: Single step duplex kDNA-PCR for detection of *Leishmania donovani* complex in human peripheral blood samples. Diagn Microbiol Infect Dis 2006;56:395–400.

22 Mary C, Faraut F, Lascombe L, Dumon H. Quantification of *Leishmania infantum* DNA by a real time PCR assay with high sensitivity. J Clin Microbiol 2004; 42:5249–5255.

23 Wortmann G, Hochberg L, Houng HH, Sweeney C, Zapor M, Aronson N, Weina P, Ockenhouse CF: Rapid identification of Leishmania complexes by a real-time PCR assay. Am J Med Hyg 2005; 73: 999–1004.

24 Castilho TM, Shaw JJ, Floeter-Winter LM: New PCR assay using glucose-6-phosphate dehydrogenase for identification of *Leishmania* species. J Clin Microbiol 2003;41:540–546.

25 Foulet F, Botterel F, Buffet P, Morizot G, Rivollet D, Deniau M, Pratlong F,Costa JM, Bretagne S: Detection and identification of *Leishmania* species from clinical specimens by using a real-time PCR assay and sequencing of the cytochrome B gene. J Clin Microbiol 2007;45:2110–2115.

26 Selvapandiyan A, Duncan R, Mendez J, Kumar R, Salotra P, Cardo LJ, Nakhasi HL: A leishmania minicircle DNA footprint assay for sensitive detection and rapid speciation of clinical isolates. Transfusion 2008;48:1787–1798.

27 Braz RF, Nascimento ET, Martins DR, Wilson ME, Pearson RD, Reed SG, Jeronimo SM: The sensitivity and specificity of *Leishmania chagasi* recombinant K39 antigen in the diagnosis of American visceral leishmaniasis and in differentiating active from subclinical infection. Am J Trop Med Hyg 2002;67:344–348.

28 Suffia I, Quaranta JF, Eulalio MC, Ferrua B, Marty P, Le Fichoux Y, Kubar J: Human T-cell activation by 14- and 18-kilodalton nuclear proteins of *Leishmania infantum*. Infect Immun 1995;63:3765–3771.

29 Bekanntmachung der Richtlinien zur Gewinnung von Blut und Blutbestandteilen und zur Anwendung von Blutprodukten (Hämotherapie) gemäß §§ 12 und 18 des Transfusionsgesetzes (TFG) (Novelle 2005) vom 19. September 2005. Bundesanzeiger 5. November 2005, Jahrgang 57, Nummer 209a.

30 Bekanntmachung der Richtlinien zur Gewinnung von Blut und Blutbestandteilen und zur Anwendung von Blutprodukten (Hämotherapie) gemäß §§ 12 und 18 des Transfusionsgesetzes (TFG) (Änderungen und Ergänzungen 2007) vom 17. April 2007. Bundesanzeiger 10. Mai 2007, Nr 92, S. 5075.

31 Reesink HW, Engelfriet CP, Wendel S, Delage G, Gao F, Tamme J, Elghouzzi MH, Laperche S, Lefrère JJ, O'Riordan JM, Shinar E, Prati D, Raffaele L, Satake M, Hernandez JM, Boukef K, LeibyDA, Stramer SL, Nakhasi H, Epstein JS: Are current measures to prevent transfusion-associated protozoal infections sufficient? Vox Sang 2004;87:125–138.

32 Matheron S, Cabié A, Parquin F, Mayaud P, Roux P, Antoine M, Chougnet C, Coulaud JP: Visceral leishmaniasis and HIV infection: unusual presentation with pleuropulmonary involvement, and effect of secondary prophylaxis. AIDS 1992;6:238–240.

33 Alvar J, Cañavate C, Gutiérrez-Solar B, Jiménez M, Laguna F, Lopez-Vélez R, Molina R, Moreno J: Leishmania and human immunodeficiency virus coinfection: the first 10 years. Clin Microbiol Rev 1997; 10:298–319.

34 Bhattacharya SK, Sinha PK, Sundar S, Thakur CP, Jha TK, Pandey K, Das VR, Kumar N, Lal C, Verma N, Singh VP, Ranjan A, Verma RB, Anders G, Sindermann H, Ganguly NK: Phase 4 trial of miltefosine for the treatment of Indian visceral Leishmaniasis. J Infect Dis 2007;196:591–598.

35 Jha TK, Sundar S, Thakur CP, Bachmann P, Karbwang J, Fischer C, Voss A, Berman J: Miltefosine, an oral agent, for the treatment of Indian visceral leishmaniasis. N Engl J Med 1999;341:1795–1800.

36 Arevalo I, Tulliano G, Quispe A, Spaeth G, Matiashewski G, Llanos-Cuentas A, Pollack H: Role of imiquimod and parenteral meglumine antimoniate in the initial treatment of cutaneous leishmaniasis. Clin Infect Dis 2007;44:1549–1554.

37 Coelho AC, Messier N, Ouelette M, Cotrim PC: Role of the ABC transporter PRP1 (ABCC7) in pentamidine resistance in *Leishmania amastigotes*. Antimicrob Agents Chemother 2007;51:3030–3032.

38 Ribeiro RR, Moura EP, Pimentel VM, Sampaio WM, Silva SM, Schettini DA, Alves CF, Melo FA, Tafuri WL, Demicheli C, Melo MN, Frezard F, Michalick SM: Reduced tissue parasite load and infectivity to sand flies in dogs naturally infected by *Leishmania chagasi* following treatment with a liposome formulation of meglumine antimoniate. Antimicrob Agents Chemother 2008;52:2564–2572.

39 Dey A, Singh S: Transfusion transmitted leishmaniasis: a case report and review of literature. Indian J Med Microbiol 2006;24:165–170.

40 Luz KG, da Silva VO, Gomes EM, Machado FC, Araujo MA, Fonseca HE, Freire TC, d'Almeida JB, Palatnik M, Palatnik-de Sousa CB: Prevalence of anti-*Leishmania donovani* antibody among Brazilian blood donors and multiple transfused hemodialysis patients. Am J Trop Med Hyg 1997;57:168–171.

41 Terry LL, Lewis JL Jr, Sessoms SM: Laboratory infection with *Leishmania donovani*: a case report. Am J Trop Med Hyg 1950;30:643–649.

42 Herwaldt BL: Laboratory-acquired parasitic infections from accidental exposures. Clin Microbiol Rev 2001;14:659–688.

43 Cardo LJ, Salata J, Harman R, Mendez J, Weina PJ: Leukodepletion filters reduce Leishmania in blood products when used at collection or at the bedside. Transfusion 2006;46:896–902.

44 Mathur P, Samantaray JC: The first probable case of platelet transfusion-transmitted visceral leishmaniasis. Transfus Med 2004;14:319–321.

45 Cervia JS, Wenz B, Ortolano GA: Leukocyte reduction's role in the attenuation of infection risks among transfusion recipients. Clin Infect Dis 2007;45:1008–1013.

46 Wagner SJ, Skripchenko A, Salata J, Cardo LJ: Photoinactivation of *Leishmania donovani infantum* in red cell suspensions by a flexible thiopyrylium sensitizer. Vox Sang 2006;91:178–180.

47 Eastman RT, Barrett LK, Dupuis K, Buckner FS, Van Voorhis WC: Leishmania inactivation in human pheresis platelets by a psoralen (amotosalen HCl) and long-wavelength ultraviolet irradiation. Transfusion 2005;45:1459–1463.

48 Cardo LJ, Rentas FJ, Ketchum L, Salata J, Harman R, Melvin W, Weina PJ, Mendez J, Reddy H, Goodrich R: Pathogen inactivation of *Leishmania donovani infantum* in plasma and platelet concentrates using riboflavin and ultraviolet light. Vox Sang 2006;90:85–91.
49 Mühlpfordt H: Vergleichende elektronenmikroskopische Untersuchung über die Markierung von *Leishmania donovani, Leishmania tropica* und *Leishmania braziliensis* mit Ferritin. Tropenmed Parasitol 1975;26:385–389.
50 Gasser RA Jr, Magill AJ, Oster CN, Tramont EC: The threat of infectious disease in Americans returning from Operation Desert Storm. N Engl J Med 1991;324:859–864.
51 Umezawa ES, Simonsen Stolf AM, Corbett CEP, Shikanai-Yasuda MA: Chagas' disease. Lancet 2000;357:797–799.
52 Chagas C: Nova tripanosomiase humana. Estudos sobre el morfolojia e o ciclo evolutivo do *Schizotrypanum cruzi* n. gen., n. sp., ajente etiolójico de nova entidade mórbida do homem – Ueber eine neue Trypanosomiasis des Menschen. Studien über Morphologie und Entwicklungszyklus des *Schizotrypanum cruzi* n. gen., n. sp., Erreger einer neuen Krankheit des Menschen. Mem Inst Oswaldo Cruz 1909;1:159–218.
53 Atkin J: The navy surgeon or a practical system of surgery. London, Caesar Ward and Richard Chandler, 1734
54 Nepveu G: Sur un trypanosome dans le sang de l'homme. Compt Rend Soc Biol (Marseille) 1898; 5:1172–1174.
55 Kirchhoff LV. Trypanosoma species (American trypanosomiasis, Chagas disease): biology of Ttrypanosomes; in Mandell GL, Benett JE, Dolin R (eds): Principles and Practice of Infectious Diseases, 6th ed. Orlando, Churchill Livingstone, 2005, pp 3156–3164.
56 Manson's Tropical Medicine, 21 ed. Amsterdam, Elsevier, 2002.
57 Crovato F, Rebora A: Chagas' disease: a potential plague for Europe? Dermatology 1997;195:184–185,
58 Jelinek T, Bisoffi Z, Bonazzi L, van Thiel P, Bronner U, de Frey A, Gundersen SG, McWhinney P, Ripamonti D; European Network on Imported Infectious Disease Surveillance: Cluster of African trypanosomiasis in travelers to Tanzanian national parks. Emerg Infect Dis 2002;8:634–635.
59 Chappuis F, Loutan L, Simarro P, Lejon V, Büscher P: Options for field diagnosis of human African trypanosomiasis. Clin Microbiol Rev 2005;18:133–146.
60 Oelemann W, Vanderborght BO, Verissimo Da Costa GC, Teixeira MG, Borges-Pereira J, De Castro JA, Coura JR, Stoops E, Hulstaert F, Zrein M, Peralta JM: A recombinant peptide antigen line immunoassay optimized for the confirmation of Chagas' disease. Transfusion 1999;39:711–717.
61 Umezawa ES, Bastos SF, Coura JR, Levin MJ, Gonzalez A, Rangel-Aldao R, Zingales B, Luquetti AO, da Silveira JF: An improved serodiagnostic test for Chagas' disease employing a mixture of *Trypanosoma cruzi* recombinant antigens. Transfusion 2003;43:91–97.
62 Roddy P, Goiri J, Flevaud L, Palma PP, Morote S, Lima N, Villa L, Torrico F, Albajar-Viñas P: Field evaluation of a rapid immunochromatographic assay for detection of *Trypanosoma cruzi* infection by use of whole blood. J Clin Microbiol 2008;46:2022–2027.
63 Jamonneau V, Solano P, Garcia A, Lejon V, Djé N, Miezan TW, N'Guessan P, Cuny G, Büscher P: Stage determination and therapeutic decision in human African trypanosomiasis: value of polymerase chain reaction and immunoglobulin M quantification on the cerebrospinal fluid of sleeping sickness patients in Côte d'Ivoire. Trop Med Int Health 2003; 8:589–594.
64 Schuster FL, Sullivan JJ: Cultivation of clinically significant hemoflagellates. Clin Microbiol Rev 2002; 15:374–389.
65 Coimbra VC, Yamamoto D, Khusal KG, Atayde VD, Fernandes MC, Mortara RA, Yoshida N, Alves MJ, Rabinovitch M: Enucleated L929 cells support invasion, differentiation and multiplication of *Trypanosoma cruzi* parasites. Infect Immun 2007;75:3700–3706.
66 Neva FA, Malone MF, Myers BR: Factors influencing the intracellular growth of *Trypanosoma cruzi* in vitro. Am J Trop Med Hyg 1961;10:140–154.
67 Novy FG, McNeal WJ: On the cultivation of *Trypanosoma brucei*. J Infect Dis 1904;1:1–30.
68 Wickstead B, Ersfeld K, Gull K: Repetitive elements in genomes of parasitic protozoa. Microbiol Mol Biol Rev 2003;67:360–375.
69 Kirchhoff LV, Votava JR, Ochs DE, Moser DR: Comparison of PCR and microscopic methods for detecting *Trypanosoma cruzi*. J Clin Microbiol 1996; 34:1171–1175.
70 Sturm NR, Degrave W, Morel C, Simpson L: Sensitive detection and schizodeme classification of *Trypanosoma cruzi* cells by amplification of kinetoplast minicircle DNA sequences: use in diagnosis of Chagas disease. Mol Biochem Parasitol 1989;33: 205–214.
71 Wincker P, Britto C, Pereira JB, Cardoso MA, Oelemann W, Morel CM: Use of a simplified polymerase chain reaction procedure to detect *Trypanosoma cruzi* in blood samples from chronic chagasic patients in a rural endemic area. Am J Trop Med Hyg 1994;51:771–777.
72 Coronado X, Zulantay I, Reyes E, Apt W, Venegas J, Rodriguez R, Solari A, Sanchez G: Comparison of *Trypanosoma cruzi* detection by PCR in blood and dejections of *Triatoma infestans* fed on patients with chronic Chagas disease. Acta Trop 2006;98:314–317.
73 Galvão LMC, Chiari E, Macedo AM, Luquetti AO, Silva SA, Andrade AL: PCR assay for monitoring *Trypanosoma cruzi* parasitemia in childhood after specific chemotherapy. J Clin Microbiol 2003;41:5066–5070.
74 Solari A, Ortiz S, Soto A, Arancibia C, Campillay R, Contreras M, Salinas P, Rojas A, Schenone H: Treatment of *Trypanosoma cruzi*-infected children with nifurtimox: a 3 year follow-up by PCR. J Antimicrob Chemother 2001;48:515–519.
75 Martins HR, Silva RM, Valadares HM, Toledo MJ, Veloso VM, Vitelli-Avelar DM, Carneiro CM, Machado-Coelho GL, Bahia MT, Martins-Filho OA, Macedo AM, Lana M: Impact of dual infections on chemotherapeutic efficacy in BALB/c mice infected with major genotypes of *Trypanosoma cruzi*. Antimicrob Agents Chemother 2007;51:3282–3289.
76 Simo G, Herder S, Njiokou F, Asonganyi T, Tilley A, Cuny G: *Trypanosoma brucei* s.l.: characterisation of stocks from Central Africa by PCR analysis of mobile genetic elements. Exp Parasitol 2005;110:353–362.
77 Becker S, Franco JR, Simarro PP, Stich A, Abel PM, Steverding D: Real-time PCR for detection of *Trypanosoma brucei* in human blood samples. Diagn Microbiol Infect Dis 2004;50:193–199.
78 Ravel S, Grébaut P, Cuisance D, Cuny G: Monitoring the developmental status of *Trypanosoma brucei gambiense* in the tsetse fly by means of PCR analysis of anal and saliva drops. Acta Trop 2003;88: 161–165.
79 Shulman IA, Appleman MD, Saxena S, Hiti AL, Kirchhoff LV: Specific antibodies to *Trypanosoma cruzi* among blood donors in Los Angeles, California. Transfusion 1997;37:727–731.
80 Leiby DA, Read EJ, Lenes BA, Yund AJ, Stumpf RJ, Kirchhoff LV, Dodd RY: Seroepidemiology of *Typanosoma cruzi*, etiologic agent of Chagas disease, in US blood donors. J Infect Dis 1997;176:1047–1052.
81 Kirchhoff LV, Paredes P, Lomeli-Guerrero A, Espinoza M, Ron-Guerrero CS, Delgado-Mejia M, Peña-Muñoz JG: Transfusion-associated Chagas disease (American trypanosomiasis) in Mexico: implications for transfusion medicine in the United States. Transfusion 2006;46:298–304.
82 Young C, Losikoff P, Chawla A, Glasser L, Forman E: Transfusion-acquired *Trypanosoma cruzi* infection. Transfusion 2007;47:540–544.
83 Centers for Disease Control and Prevention (CDC): Chagas disease after organ transplantation – Los Angeles, California 2006. MMWR Morb Mortal Wkly Rep 2006;55:798–800.
84 Villalba R, Fornés G, Alvarez MA, Román J, Rubio V, Fernández M, Garcia JM, Viñals M, Torres A: Acute Chagas' disease in a recipient of a bone marrow transplant in Spain: case report. Clin Infect Dis 1992;14:594–595.
85 Schmunis GA, Cruz JR: Safety of the blood supply in Latin America. Clin Microbiol Rev 2005;18: 12–29.
86 O'Brien SFO, Chiavetta JA, Fan W, Xi G, Yi QL, Goldman M, Scalia V, Fearon MA: Assessment of a travel question to identify donors with risk of *Trypanosoma cruzi*: operational validity and field testing. Transfusion 2008;48:755–761.
87 Leiby DA, Herron RM, Garratty G, Herwaldt BL: *Trypanosoma cruzi* parasitemia in US blood donors with serologic evidence of infection. J Infect Dis 2008; 198:609–613.
88 Frank M, Hegenscheid B, Janitschke K, Weinke T: Prevalence and epidemiological significance of *Trypanosoma cruzi* infection among Latin American immigrants in Berlin, Germany. Infection 1997;25:355–358.
89 Olivares-Illiana V, Rodriguez-Romero A, Becker I, Berzunza M, Garcia J, Pérez-Montfort R, Cabrera N, López-Calahorra F, de Gómez-Puyou MT, Gomez-Puyou A: Perturbation of the dimer interface of triosephosphate isomerase and its effect on trypanosoma cruzi. PLOS Negl Trop Dis 2007;1: e01-e08.
90 Uzcátegui NL, Carmona-Gutierrez D, Denninger V, Schoenfeld C, Lang F, Figarella K, Duszenko M: Antiproliferative effect of dihydroxyacetone on *Trypanosoma brucei* bloodstream forms: cell cycle progression, subcellular alterations, and cell death. Antimicrob Agents Chemother 2007;51:3960–3968.
91 Lejon V, Roger I, Ngoyi DM, Menten J, Robays J, N'Siesi FX, Bisser S, Boelaert M, Büscher P: Novel markers for treatment outcome in late stage *Trypanosoma brucei gambiense* trypanosomiasis. Clin Infect Dis 2008;47:15–22.
92 Castro E, Gironés N, Bueno JL, Carrión J, Lin L, Fresno M: The efficacy of photochemical treatment with amotosalen HCl and ultraviolet A (Intercept) for inactivation of *Trypanosoma cruzi* in pooled buffy-coat platelets. Transfusion 2007;47:434–441.

93 Gelfand JA, Vannier E: Babesia species; in Mandell GL, Benett JE, Dolin R (eds): Principles and Practice of Infectious Diseases, 6th ed. Orlando, Churchill Livingstone, 2005, pp 3209–3215.
94 White DJ, Talarico J, Chang HG, Birkhead GS, Heimberger T, Morse DL: Human babesiosis in New York State: review of 139 hospitalized cases and analysis of prognostic factors. Arch Intern Med 1998;158:2149–2154.
95 Hilpertshauser H, Deplazes P, Schnyder M, Gern L, Mathis A: *Babesia* spp. identified by PCR in ticks collected from domestic and wild ruminants in southern Switzerland. Appl Environ Microbiol 2006;72:6503–6507.
96 Gorenflot A, Moubri K, Precigout E, Carcy B, Schetters TP: Human babesiosis. Ann Trop Med Parasitol 1998;92:489–501.
97 Kjemtrup AM, Conrad PA: Human babesiosis: an emerging tick-borne disease. Int J Parasitol 2000;30:1323–1337.
98 Olmeda AS, Armstrong PM, Rosenthal BM, Valladares B, del Castillo A, de Armas F, Miguelez M, Gonzalez A, Rodriguez JA, Spielman A, Telford SR 3rd: A subtropical case of human babesiosis. Acta Trop 1997;67:229–234.
99 Häselbarth K, Tenter AM, Brade V, Krieger G, Hunfeld KP: First case of human babesiosis in Germany – clinical presentation and molecular characterisation of the pathogen. Int J Med Microbiol 2007;297:197–204.
100 Hartelt K, Oehme R, Frank H, Brockmann SO, Hassler D, Kimmig P: Pathogens and symbionts in ticks: prevalence of *Anaplasma phagocytophilum* (*Ehrlichia* sp.), *Wolbachia* sp., *Rickettsia* sp. and *Babesia* sp. in Southern Germany. Int J Med Microbiol 2004;293(suppl 37):86–92.
101 Heile C, Heydorn AO, Schein E: *Dermatocentor reticulatus* (Fabricius, 1794) – Verbreitung, Biologie und Vektor für *Babesia canis* in Deutschland. Berl Münch Tierärztl Wochenschr 2006;119: 330–334.
102 Máthé A, Vörös K, Papp L, Reiczigel J: Clinical manifestations of canine babesiosis in Hungary (63 cases). Acta Vet Hung 2006;54:367–385.
103 Hunfeld KP, Lambert A, Kampen H, Albert S, Epe C, Brade V, Tenter AM: Seroprevalence of Babesia infections in humans exposed to ticks in midwestern Germany. J Clin Microbiol 2002; 40:2431–2436.
104 Foppa IM, Krause PJ, Spielman A, Goethert H, Gern L, Brand B, Telford SR 3rd: Entomologic and serologic evidence of zoonotic transmission of *Babesia microti*, eastern Switzerland. Emerg Infect Dis 2002;8:722–726.
105 Boustani MR, Gelfand JA: Babesiosis. Clin Infect Dis 1996;22:611–615.
106 Schuster FL: Cultivation of Babesia and Babesia-like blood parasites: agents of an emerging zoonotic disease. Clin Microbiol Rev 2002;15:365–373.
107 Grande N, Precigout E, Ancelin ML, Moubri K, Carcy B, Lemesre JL, Vial H, Gorenflot A: Continuous in vitro culture of *Babesia divergens* in a serum-free medium. Parasitology 1997;115:81–89.
108 Persing DH, Mathiesen D, Marshall WF, Telford SR 3rd, Spielman A, Thomford JW, Conrad PA: Detection of *Babesia microti* by polymerase chain reaction. J Clin Microbiol 1992;30:2097–2103.
109 Krause PJ, Telford S 3rd, Spielman A, Ryan R, Magera J, Rajan TV, Christianson D, Alberghini TV, Bow L, Persing D: Comparison of PCR with blood smear and inoculation of small animals for diagnosis of *Babesia microti* parasitemia. J Clin Microbiol 1996;34:2791–2794.
110 Krause PJ, Spielman A, Telford SR 3rd, Sikand VK, McKay K, Christianson D, Pollack RJ, Brassard P, Magera J, Ryan R, Persing DH: Persistent parasitaemia after acute babesiosis. N Engl J Med 1998;339:160–165.
111 Shayan P, Rahbari S: Simultaneous differentiation between *Theileria* spp. and *Babesia* spp. on stained blood smear using PCR. Parasitol Res 2005;97: 281–286.
112 Krampitz HE, Buschmann H, Münchoff P: Gibt es latente Babesien-Infektionen beim Menschen in Süddeutschland? Mitt Österr Ges Tropenmed Parasitol 1986;8:233–243.
113 Leiby DA, Chung AP, Cable RG, Trouern-Trend J, McCullough J, Homer MJ, Reynolds LD, Houghton RL, Lodes MJ, Persing DH: Relationship between tick bites and the seroprevalence of *Babesia microti* and *Anaplasma phagocytophila* (previously *Ehrlichia* sp.) in blood donors. Transfusion 2002;42:1585–1591.
114 Leiby DA, Chung AP, Gill JE, Houghton RL, Persing DH, Badon S, Cable RG: Demonstrable parasitemia among Connecticut blood donors with antibodies to *Babesia microti*. Transfusion 2005; 45:1804–1810.
115 Grabowski EF, Giardina PJ, Goldberg D, Masur H, Read SE, Hirsch RL, Benach JL: Babesiosis transmitted by a transfusion of frozen-thawed blood. Ann Intern Med 1982;96:466–467.
116 Marcus LC, Valigorsky JM, Fanning WL, Joseph T, Glick B: A case report of transfusion induced babesiosis. JAMA 1982;248:465–467.
117 Mintz ED, Anderson JF, Cable RG, Hadler JL· Transfusion-transmitted babesiosis: a case report from a new endemic area. Transfusion 1991;31: 365–368.
118 Popovsky MA: Transfusion-transmitted babesiosis. Transfusion 1991;31:296–298.
119 Homer MJ, Aguilar-Delfin I, Telford SR 3rd, Krause PJ, Persing DH: Babesiosis. Clin Microbiol Rev 2000;13:451–469.
120 Kain KC, Jassoum SB, Fong IW, Hannach B: Transfusion-transmitted babesiosis in Ontario: first reported case in Canada. CMAJ 2001;164: 1721–1723.
121 Herwaldt BL, Neitzel DF, Gorlin JB, Jensen KA, Perry EH, Peglow WR, Slemenda SB, Won KY, Nace EK, Pieniazek NJ, Wilson M: Transmission of *Babesia microti* in Minnesota through four blood donations from the same donor over a 6-month period. Transfusion 2002;42:1154–1158.
122 New DL, Quinn JB, Qureshi MZ, Sigler SJ: Vertically transmitted babesiosis. J Pediatr 1997;131: 163–164.
123 Lux JZ, Weiss D, Linden JV, Kessler D, Herwaldt BL, Wong SJ, Keithly J, Della-Latta P, Scully BE: Transfusion-associated babesiosis after heart transplant. Emerg Infec Dis 2003;9:116–119.
124 Gupta P, Hurley RW, Helseth PH, Goodman JL, Hammerschmidt DE: Pancytopenia due to hemophagocytic syndrome as the presenting manifestation of babesiosis. Am J Hematol 1995;50:60–62.
125 Slovut DP, Benedetti E, Matas AJ: Babesiosis and hemophagocytic syndrome in a asplenic transplant recipient. Transplantation 1996;62:537–539.
126 Perdrizet GA, Olson NH, Krause PJ, Banever GT, Spielman A, Cable RG: Babesiosis in a renal transplant recipient acquired through blood transfusion. Transplantation 2000;70:205–208.
127 Callow LL, Dagliesh RJ, de Vos AJ: Development of effective living vaccines against bovine babesiosis – the longest field trial? Int J Parasitol 1997;27:747–767.
128 Ushe TC, Palmer GH, Sotomayor L, Figueroa JV, Buening GM, Perryman LE, McElwain TF: Antibody reponse to a *Babesia bigemina* rhoptry-associated protein 1 surface-exposed and neutralization sensitive epitope in immune cattle. Infect Immun 1994;62:5698–5701.
129 Berens SJ, Brayton KA, Molloy JB, Bock RE, Lew AE, McElwain TF: Merozoite surface antigen 2 proteins of Babesia bovis vaccine breakthrough isolates contain a unique hypervariable region composed of degenerate repeats. Infect Immun 2005; 73:7180–7189.
130 Leroith T, Brayton KA, Molloy JB, Bock RE, Hines SA, Lew AE, McElwain TF: Sequence variation and immunologic cross-reactivity among *Babesia bovis* merozoite surface antigen 1 proteins from vaccine strains and vaccine breakthrough isolates. Infect Immun 2005;73:5388–5394.
131 Gerber MA, Shapiro ED, Krause PJ, Cable RG, Badon SJ, Ryan RW: The risk of acquiring Lyme disease or babesiosis from a blood tranfusion. J Infect Dis 1994;170:231–234.
132 Singh Y, Sawyer LS, Pinkoski LS, Dupuis KW, Hsu JC, Lin L, Corash L: Photochemical treatment of plasma with amotosalen and long-wavelength ultraviolet light inactivates pathogens while retaining coagulation function. Transfusion 2006;46: 1168–1177.
133 Holman PJ, Waldrup KA, Wagner GG: In vitro cultivation of a Babesia isolated from a white-tailed deer (*Odocoileus virginianus*). J Parasitol 1988;74:111–115.
134 Canning EU, Winger CM. Babesidiae; in Taylor AER, Baker JR (eds): In vitro Methods for Parasite Cultivation. New York, Academic Press, 1987, pp 199–229.
135 Nicolle C, Manceaux L: Sur un protozoaire nouveau du gondi, Toxoplasma. Arch Inst Pasteur Tunis 1909;2:97–103.
136 Splendore A: Sur un nouveau protozoaire parasite du lapin, deuxième note préliminaire. Bull Soc Pathol Exot 1909;2:462–465.
137 Wolf A, Cowen D: Granulomatous encephalomyelitis due to an encephalitozoon (encephalitozoic encephalomyelitis). A new protozoon disease of man. Bull Neurol Inst New York 1937;6:306–371.
138 Montoya JG, Kovacs JA, Remington JS: *Toxoplasma gondii*; in Mandell GL, Benett JE, Dolin R (eds): Principles and Practice of Infectious Diseases, 6th ed. Orlando, Churchill Livingstone, 2005, pp 3170–3198
139 Fuentes I, Rubio JM, Ramirez C, Alvar J: Genotypic characterization of *Toxoplasma gondii* strains associated with human toxoplasmosis in Spain: direct analysis from clinical samples. J Clin Microbiol 2001;39:1566–1570.
140 Howe DK, Honoré S, Derouin F, Sibley LD: Determination of genotypes of *Toxoplasma gondii* strains isolated from patients with toxoplasmosis. J Clin Microbiol 1997;35:1411–1414.
141 Dubey JP: Advances in the life cycle of *Toxoplasma gondii*. Int J Parasitol 1998;28:1019–1024.
142 Ferguson DJ, Hutchison WM, Pettersen E: Tissue cyst rupture in mice chronically infected with *Toxoplasma gondii*. Parasitol Res 1989;75:599–603.
143 Hill D, Dubey JP: *Toxoplasma gondii*: transmission, diagnosis and prevention. Clin Microbiol Infect 2002;8:634–640.
144 Remington JS, Cavanaugh EN: Isolation of the endocysted form of *Toxoplasma gondii* from human skeletal muscle and brain. N Engl J Med 1965;273:1308–1310.

145 Suzuki Y, Orellana MA, Schreiber RD, Remington JS: Interferon-gamma: the major mediator of resistance against *Toxoplasma gondii*. Science 1988;240: 516–518.
146 Suzuki Y, Wong SY, Grumet FC, Fessel J, Montoya JG, Zolopa AR, Portmore A, Schumacher-Perdreau F, Schrappe M, Köppen S, Ruf B, Brown BW, Remington JS: Evidence for genetic regulation of susceptibility to toxoplasmic encephalitis in AIDS patients. J Infect Dis 1996;173:265–268.
147 Swartzberg JE, Remington JS: Transmission of Toxoplasma. Am J Dis Child 1975;129:777–779.
148 Krauss H, Weber A, Appel M, Enders B, Isenberg HD, Schieder HG, Slenczka W, von Graevenitz A, Zahner H: Zoonoses. Infectious Diseases Transmissible from Animals to Humans. 3rd ed, Washington, ASM Press, 2003, pp 307–308.
149 Heu HC:. Toxoplasmosis transmitted at autopsy. J Am Med Ass 1967;202:284–285.
150 Clumeck N: Some aspects of the epidemiology of toxoplasmosis and pneumocystosis in AIDS in Europe. Eur J Clin Microbiol Dis 1991;10:177–178.
151 Zumla A, Savva D, Wheeler RB, Hira SK, Luo NP, Kaleebu P, Sempala SK, Johnson JD, Holliman R: Toxoplasma serology in Zambian and Ugandan patients infected with the human immunodeficiency virus. Trans R Soc Trop Med Hyg 1991;85:227–229.
152 Belanger F, Derouin F, Grangeat-Keros L, Meyer L, Hemoco and Seroco Study Groups: Incidence and risk factors of toxoplasmosis in a cohort of human immunodeficiency virus-infected patients: 1988–1995. Clin Infect Dis 1999;28: 575–581.
153 Rilling V, Dietz K, Krczal D, Knotek F, Enders G: Evaluation of a commercial IgG/IgM Western blot assay for early postnatal diagnosis of congenital toxoplasmosis. Eur J Clin Microbiol Infect Dis 2003;22:174–180.
154 Franck J, Garin YJF, Dumon H: LDBio-Toxo II Immunoglobulin western blot confirmatory test for anti-toxoplasma antibody detection. J Clin Microbiol 2008;46:2334–2338.
155 Nielsen HV, Schmidt DR, Petersen E: Diagnosis of congenital toxoplasmosis by two-dimensional immunoblot differentiation of mother and child immunoglobulin G profiles. J Clin Microbiol 2005;43: 711–715.
156 Kodym P, Machala L, Roháčová H, Sirocká B, Maly M: Evaluation of a commercial IgE ELISA in comparison with IgA and IgM ELISAs, IgG avidity assay and complement fixation for the diagnosis of acute toxoplasmosis. Clin Microbiol Infect 2007; 13:40–47.
157 Liesenfeld O, Press C, Montoya JG, Gill R, Isaac-RentonJL, Hedman K, Remington JS: False-positive results in immunoglobulin M (IgM) toxoplasma antibody tests and importance of confirmatory testing: the Platelia Toxo IgM test. J Clin Microbiol 1997;35:174–178.
158 Foudrinier F, Villena I, Jaussaud R, Aubert D, Chemla C, Martinot F, Pinon JM: Clinical value of specific immunoglobulin E detection by enzyme-linked immunosorbent assay in cases of acquired and congenital toxoplasmosis. J Clin Microbiol 2003; 41:1681–1686.
159 Saad R, Vincent JF, Cimon B, de Gentile F, Francois S, Bouachour G, Ifrah N: Pulmonary toxoplasmosis after allogeneic bone marrow transplantation: case report and review. Bone Marrow Transplant 1996;18:211–212.
160 Van Knapen F, Panggabean SO: Detection of toxoplasma antigen in tissues by means of enzyme-linked immunosorbent assay (ELISA). Am J Clin Pathol 1982;77:755–757.
161 Frenkel JK, Piekarski G: The demonstration of Toxoplasma and other organisms by immunofluorescence: a pitfall (Editorial). J Infect Dis 1978;138: 265–266.
162 Cinque P, Scarpellini P, Vago L, Linde A, Lazzarin A: Diagnosis of central nervous system complications in HIV-infected patients: cerebrospinal fluid analysis by the polymerase chain reaction. AIDS 1997;11:1–17.
163 Dupouy-Camet J, de Souza SL, Maslo C, Paugam A, Saimot AG, Benarous R, Tourte-Schaefer C, Derouin F: Detection of *Toxoplasma gondii* in venous blood from AIDS patients by polymerase chain reaction. J Clin Microbiol 1993;31: 1866–1869.
164 Costa JM, Pautas C, Ernault P, Foulet F, Cordonnier C, Bretagne S: Real-time PCR for diagnosis and follow up of Toxoplasma reactivation after allogeneic stem cell transplantation using fluorescence resonance energy transfer hybridization probes. J Clin Microbiol 2000;38:2929–2932.
165 Remington JS, Thulliez P, Montoya JG: Recent developments for diagnosis of toxoplasmosis. J Clin Microbiol 2004;42:941–945.
166 Ajzenberg D, Dumètre A, Dardé ML: Multiplex PCR for typing strains of Toxoplasma gondii. J Clin Microbiol 2005;43:1940–1943.
167 Calderaro A, Piccolo G, Gorrini C, Peruzzi S, Zerbini L, Bommezzardi S, Dettori G, Chezzi C: Comparison between two real-time PCR assays and a nested-PCR for the detection of *Toxoplasma gondii*. Acta Biomed 2006;77:75–80.
168 Joss AW, Evans R, Mavin S, Chatterton J, Ho-Yen DO: Development of real-time PCR to detect *Toxoplasma gondii* and *Borrelia burgdorferi* infections in postal samples. J Clin Pathol 2008;61:221–224.
169 Goebel WS, Conway JH, Faught P, Vakili ST, Haut PR: Disseminated toxoplasmosis resulting in graft failure in a cord blood stem cell transplant recipient. Pediatr Blood Cancer 2007;48:222–226.
170 Pinlaor S, Leamviteevanich K, Pinlaor P, Maleewong W, Pipitgool V: Seroprevalence of specific total immunoglobulin (Ig) IgG and IgM antibodies to *Toxoplasma gondii* in blood donors from Loei Province, Northeast Thailand. Southeast Asian J Trop Med Public Health 2000;31:123–127.
171 Jacquier P, Nadal D, Zuber P, Eckert J: The status of infection with *Toxoplasma gondii* in the Swiss population: contribution of a seroepidemiologic study from the Zurich canton. Schweiz Med Wochenschr Suppl 1995;65:23S–28S.
172 Levy JA: HIV and the Pathogenesis of AIDS, 3rd ed. Washington, ASM – American Society of Microbiology, 2007.
173 Assi MA, Rosenblatt JE, Marshall WF: Donor-transmitted toxoplasmosis in liver transplant recipients: a case report and literature review. Transpl Infect Dis 2007;9:132–136.
174 Leal FE, Cavazzana CL, de Andrade HF Jr, Galisteo AJ Jr, de Mendoça JS, Kallas EG: *Toxoplasma gondii* pneumonia in immunocompetent subjects: case report and review. Clin Infect Dis 2007;44: e62–e66.
175 Cibickova L, Horacek J, Prasil P, Slovacek L, Kohout A, Cerovsky V, Hobza V: Cerebral toxoplasmosis in an allogeneic peripheral stem cell transplant recipient: case report and review of literature. Transplant Infect Dis 2007;9:332–335.
176 Siegel SE, Lunde MN, Gelderman AH, Halterman RH, Brown JA, Levine AS, Graw RG Jr: Transmission of toxoplasmosis by leukocyte transfusion. Blood 1971;37:388–394.
177 Ryning FW, McLeod R, Maddox JC, Hunt S, Remington JS·: Probable transmission of *Toxoplasma gondii* by organ transplantation. Ann Intern Med 1979;90:47–49.
178 Martino R, Bretagne S, Rovira M, Ullmann AJ, Maertens J, Held T, Deconinck E, Cordonnier C: Toxoplasmosis after hematopoietic stem cell transplantation: Report of a 5-year survey from the Infectious Diseases Working Party of the European Group for Blood and Marrow Transplantation. Bone Marrow Transplant 2000;25:1111–1114.
179 Dubey J, Kotula A, Sharar A, Andrews CD, Lindsay DS: Effect of high temperature on infectivity of *Toxoplasma gondii* tissue cysts in pork. J Parasitol 1990;76:201–204.

Transfusion Medicine
and Hemotherapy

Transfus Med Hemother 2009;36:32–39
DOI: 10.1159/000197314

Influenza Virus

Arbeitskreis Blut, Untergruppe «Bewertung Blutassoziierter Krankheitserreger»

1 Current Knowledge about the Pathogen

1.1 Characteristics of Influenza Viruses

Influenza viruses are members of the family Orthomyxoviridae. This family represents enveloped viruses the genome of which consists of segmented negative-sense single-strand RNA segments. There are four genera of this family: types A, B, C and Thogotovirus, of which, however, only genera A and B are clinically relevant for humans. The eight genome segments of influenza A and B viruses are loosely encapsidated by the nucleoprotein. The polymerase complexes consisting of the three polymerase proteins PB1, PB2, and PA are located at the ends of the nucleocapsids. These helical capsids are encircled by the M1 matrix protein and by a host-derived lipid bilayer envelope in which the virus surface glycoproteins haemagglutinin (HA) and neuraminidase (NA) as well as the M2 matrix protein are embedded [1]. The HA is synthesized as precursor protein and cleaved by cellular serine proteases into the functional proteins HA1 and HA2. The amino acid sequence at the cleavage site determines HA processing by cellular proteases and thus, also the organ tropism. Mutations at the cleavage site of avian influenza viruses may lead to an insertion of alkaline amino acids. Ubiquitous proteases such as furin can cleave such a mutated HA and, as a consequence, permit systemic spreading of the virus. This mechanism changes a lowly pathogenic into a highly pathogenic avian influenza virus and has been associated so far only with subtype H5 and H7 viruses.

Influenza virus as an enveloped virus is relatively vulnerable to damaging environmental impacts. Depending on environmental conditions (e.g. humidity and temperature), however, it can survive up to several hours and in water at low temperatures (e.g. <20 °C) also considerably longer (up to several months). Influenza viruses are sensitive to lipid solvents and detergents. They are also vulnerable to heat and a low pH, depending on the virus type. Influenza A viruses with uncleaved HA are obviously more stable (loss of infectivity at pH <4.5) than viruses with cleaved HA (loss of infectivity at pH <5) [2].

The most outstanding characteristic of influenza viruses is their rapid evolution which leads to its great variability. This is the case especially with influenza A viruses. According to the antigenic properties of their envelope proteins, influenza A viruses are subdivided into a number of subtypes. 16 different HA and 9 different NA subtypes have been identified so far. The nomenclature system follows the pattern H(x)N(y) including the host of origin, geographical location, strain number, and year of isolation [1, 3]. Influenza B viruses are not further divided into subtypes. The accumulation of point mutations leads to a step-by-step modification of the virus proteins (above all in the two surface antigens HA and NA). This mechanism is described as 'antigen drift' and is also typical of influenza B viruses. The variability of the type B viruses, however, is also characterised by other mechanisms such as insertion and deletion, as the influenza B lines show which have been co-circulating and stable for more than 20 years [4, 5].

The process of 'antigen shift' (re-assortment) is defined as the exchange of whole genome segments, above all HA genes, which might result in influenza viruses which have a selective advantage compared with their parent viruses. A prerequisite for this re-assortment is simultaneous infection of a cell by two different influenza A viruses. This will result in a variety of different hybrid viruses with different characteristics which they have received from the parent viruses via the individual genome segments. An example is the occurrence of the influenza A/H2N2 subtype in 1957 which superseded the influenza A/H1N1 virus which was dominant until then [6, 7].

Special attention was drawn to the public by the deaths caused in humans by the highly pathogenic avian influenza A/H5N1 subtype. These cases have shown that an entirely new influenza A virus can cause deadly infections in humans. Since the first outbreaks of H5N1-related avian influenza in poultry in South-East Asia in 2003, human H5N1 transmissions with

KARGER

Fax +49 761 4 52 07 14
Information@Karger.de
www.karger.com

Accessible online at:
www.karger.com/tmh

Previously published in Transfus Med Hemother 2008;35:42–49

high mortality have occurred in 10 countries. [8]. It is possible that this virus will adapt better to humans and will then be able to spread among the human population.

1.2 Infection and Infectious Disease

Influenza viruses are assumed to be transmitted predominantly by aerosol infection, i.e. relatively large droplets (>5 µm) created particularly while talking, coughing, or sneezing, thus entering the mucosae through contact at small distances. Individual publications, however, have also suggested that transmission might occur by so-called droplet cores which are smaller (<5 µm) and able to remain in the air for longer periods (aerogenic transmission). In addition, transmission can occur by direct contact with virus-contaminated surfaces (e.g. shaking hands) and subsequent mouth-nose contact. After infection the viruses replicate in the nasal and laryngeal mucosae. This replication also affects the lower airways as the infection progresses.

A clinical characteristic of human influenza is a sudden rise in body temperature to >38.5 °C 1–3 days following infection. Other symptoms include headache, limb ache, tiredness, general faintness and dry cough. Infectivity can start already shortly (<24 h) before the onset of the clinical symptoms and usually persists 3–5 days. Small children can excrete the viruses earlier and over a longer period of time than adults. The most serious outcomes are peracute death within only few hours and primary influenza pneumonia. Encephalitis or myocarditis can also occur. Serious and fatal outcomes with primary viral and viral-bacterial pneumonia are known and have been communicated in single case reports in children and young adults [9, 10]. Complications occur particularly in older patients with primary disease (chronic heart or lung disease, metabolic disorders such as diabetes, immune disorders etc.). Such cases, above all, can involve pneumonia by bacterial superinfection (e.g. *Streptococcus pneumoniae*, *Haemophilus influenzae, Staphylococcus aureus*) [11, 12]. In children, administering salicylates may lead to Reye syndrome. Reye syndrome describes an acute cerebral function disorder. The latter occurs as a result to liver damage, usually in connection with the ingestion of acetylsalicylic acid after febrile virus infections.

The situation is different with infections of humans with avian influenza virus of the H5N1 subtype which has been circulating among the wild fowl population in South-East Asia since 2003, but also in the Middle East, in Central Africa and in South and Central Europe since autumn 2005. After a prolonged incubation period of up to 7 days, also here the characteristic initial symptoms were acute rise in body temperature (>38 °C) and influenza-like symptoms, but the respiratory tract was not involved in all patients. Frequently observed symptoms included watery diarrhoea, vomiting and pain in the abdomen and the chest. Also the occurrence of encephalitis was often described. Thus, an infection of tissues outside the respiratory tract occurs so that short-term viraemia has to be assumed (cf. 4.1). This could be confirmed by laboratory diagnosis in the case of the fatal outcome of an H5N1 infection in a boy in Thailand [13]. Taken together, the course of the disease is extremely aggressive, resulting in rapid worsening of the patient's condition and a high mortality rate [14, 15].

1.3 Epidemiology

While influenza B infections occur only in humans, influenza A viruses can also infect pigs and horses. Wild birds, above all water fowl, in which all HA and NA types occur are considered as a reservoir for influenza A viruses [16, 17]. Infections with the so-called highly pathogenic subtypes H5 and H7 can occur in chickens but also other types of birds and cause the clinical picture of classical avian plague (highly pathogenic avian influenza; HPAI), often also called bird flu. The cause for this is that the virus can replicate throughout the bird's body, resulting in disease with a high mortality rate.

Since 1977, a co-circulation of the subtypes influenza A/H3N2 and A/H1N1 as well as influenza B can be observed in humans. Human viruses of the subtype H1N2 were first observed sporadically in 1977, but not in the following years until the season of 2001/2002, when they caused local outbreaks in some countries. These viruses, however, did not become epidemiologically significant and have not been identified since 2005 [18].

Human influenza virus infections have a world-wide distribution. Seasonal influenza epidemics occur regularly both in the Northern and the Southern hemispheres each winter. Due to the seasonal shift, the winter influenza outbreak of the Southern hemisphere occurs during the summer of the Northern hemisphere. These influenza epidemics are estimated to cause approximately 500,000 deaths per year world-wide [19]. Little is known about the epidemiology of influenza in tropical countries, but it is assumed that influenza can occur throughout the year there.

Despite the pronounced seasonal dependency, influenza infections in the respective countries can also occur outside the normal influenza epidemics and can even lead to locally and temporally limited outbreaks. During the annual influenza epidemics, an estimated rate of 10–15% of the population is affected. The influenza epidemics can also be clearly distinguished from each other by the degree of severity. National influenza surveillance in Germany rests on three pillars: identification and characterization of circulating viruses by the Nationales Referenzzentrum für Influenza (National Reference Centre for Influenza) at the Robert Koch-Institut, the sentinel system of the Arbeitsgemeinschaft Influenza (AGI; Influenza Working Party) and the obligation to report the identification of virus by diagnostics in the laboratory. In the past few years, the seasons of 2002/2003 and 2004/2005 were characterised by extraordinarily high influenza virus activity. During the period of 2000/2001 to 2004/2005, the annual influenza outbreaks caused approximately 2,900,000 excess consultations, 900,000 sick notes among the working population (estimated for the age groups 16–60 years), 14,000 additional hospitalisations, and approximately 10,000 deaths compared with the periods without influenza virus circulation [20, 21]. The majority of influenza-associated deaths concerns the age group of the over 60-year-olds, not only in Germany but also in other countries [20, 22].

Influenza pandemics are characterised by the occurrence (recurrence) of influenza A subtype against which the majority of the human population is not immune, thus causing a worldwide epidemic. The past century was characterised by three major pandemics: The Spanish Flu of 1918 (H1N1) caused about 40 million deaths, while the death rates of Asian influenza of 1957 (H2N2) and Hong Kong Flu of 1968 (H2N3) were estimated at 1–2 million and 0.75–1 million deaths, respectively [19].

Special public attention was paid to the outbreak of classical avian influenza in the Netherlands and Belgium in spring 2003 by influenza A H7N7, and the influenza A H5N1 epidemic which started in South-East Asia in 1998, because they also affected humans. It is suspected that the next pandemic could also be caused by the highly pathogenic influenza virus of the H5N1 subtype. Up to now, the virus has circulated exclusively in (wild) birds. Humans have been infected only in isolated cases. Since the first human H5N1 outbreaks in 2003, 331 cases of infection and 202 deaths due to H5N1 have been officially confirmed by the WHO (data as of October 12, 2007). It is the age group of the patients that strikes us here, since mainly adolescents and young adults were affected. At present, two endemic areas with recurrent human infections and deaths have formed: Indonesia and Egypt. A genetic predisposition has been discussed since outbreaks within a family affected mainly consanguineous relatives.

1.4 Detection Methods and Their Significance

A number of methods are available for the direct detection of an influenza virus infection. As a rule, these methods use clinical materials of the upper respiratory tract (nose, pharynx), and, if indicated, e.g. in case of H5N1, also the lower respiratory tract. Serological methods now play a subordinate role in diagnosing acute infection.

1.4.1 Serology

Influenza virus-specific antibodies in the serum can be determined as total antibody levels or differentiated as single antibody sub-classes (IgA, IgM, IgG). Methods traditionally used include complement-binding reaction (CBR) and the methods preferably used today such as enzyme immunoassay (EIA) and immunofluorescence test (IFT). More sophisticated methods such as the haemagglutination inhibition test (HIT) and the neutralisation test require specialised reagents and are performed by only few laboratories in Germany. These tests can also provide information about the variant of the virus that caused the infection. An influenza virus infection will result in an IgG titre which persists for decades, but also a CBR titre can be increased during a longer period of time. Therefore, paired serum samples (at the onset of the disease and 10–14 days after the onset of the disease) should be examined for verification of an acute infection. A four-fold increase in the titre is rated as positive verification of the disease. Isolated IgA or IgG detections, however, are only of limited informational value. For both any decisions on treatment and patient management, the results of the antibody determinations would be available too late. Hence, serological methods used to identify an infection are of significance above all for epidemiological studies, for examining the effectiveness of the vaccination or for clarifying outbreaks of the infection. As far as avian influenza is concerned, however, serology is of greater significance. A reliable detection of avian influenza virus such as A/H5N1 is not always possible by means of PCR or virus culture, since it depends above all on the time when the sample is taken and the degree of severity of the disease (*www.who.int/csr/don/2006_09_14/en/index.html*). The HIT which is very well suited for human influenza detection is not sensitive enough to detect avian influenza viruses. The gold standard here is the virus neutralisation test.

1.4.2 Virus Culture

Because of the technical requirements, isolation of influenza virus is carried out in specialised laboratories only under biosafety level 2 conditions. Virus culture is very time-consuming and requires the presence of replication-competent virus particles in the patient sample. Embryonated hen eggs have been used for culturing for decades. This method is still absolutely necessary for culturing reference strains even though cell cultures have been used for primary culturing in the past few years. Madin-Darby canine kidney (MDCK) cells have proven to be particularly suitable. The appearance of a cytopathic effect can require from several days up to 2 weeks. Following this, the culture must be verified by a specific test (ELISA or IFT). To speed up the process, i.e. before the appearance of a cytopathic effect, virus-specific antigen can be detected using IFT (shell vial technique). These rapid culturing methods can produce results after 1–2 days, but are less sensitive. Virus culturing therefore plays a role neither in an out-patient nor in a hospital setting for the reasons mentioned above.

As far as national and world-wide influenza virus monitoring is concerned, however, virus culturing is of basic significance. The German National Reference Centre for Influenza is the competent authority for a comprehensive characterisation of influenza viruses circulating in Germany. The isolated viruses are examined using a panel of specific immunosera in order to determine their similarity with vaccine strains and influenza viruses circulating during the past season. In addition, molecular and phylogenetic analyses are performed in order to obtain detailed insights into the evolution of the influenza viruses and ongoing drift events [23, 24]. There is a close collaboration, both at a European level and with WHO institutions, in order to be able to make optimal recommendations on the vaccine compositions for the forthcoming season on the basis of these joint monitoring and analysis data [25].

1.4.3 Antigen Detection

Compared with virus culturing, antigen detection tests can be performed faster in any laboratory. For this purpose, commercial tests are available, e.g. IFT or ELISA. These methods provide relatively good results if there is a sufficient amount of virus antigen available in the patient's sample. The IFT is valid only if suitable sample material is available which has to be evaluated by experienced personnel. Methods such as IFT and ELISA can provide results in only a few hours. Specificity of these tests is usually very good but sensitivity is lower than with methods which either detect the virus itself or the viral genome [26–28].

Antigen tests called 'rapid tests' are available for several years. Rapid tests currently available in Germany are EIAs, which somewhat differ both in their format and in the test method. In general, the results can be obtained in approximately 10–15 min. With the exception of one test, they are all able to distinguish between influenza A and B. They are all characterised by high specificity. Data on sensitivity differ between 60 and 100% in samples of clinically ill individuals. Virus culturing and/or IFT were predominantly used as reference method. Sensitivity of these rapid tests can be compared to that of IFT and EIA [29, 30].

1.4.4 Genome Detection

Polymerase chain reaction (PCR) is a very sensitive and specific method. With the aid of specific oligonucleotide primers, the required genome sequences are replicated (amplified) in such a way that they can subsequently be detected using various techniques. Previous assays were limited to the use of primers and the analysis of the PCR product in agarose gel [31, 32]. Higher specificity of PCR, however, can be obtained by using specific probes by means of hybridisation blot [33, 34] or PCR-EIA [35, 36]. Higher specificity can also be obtained by nested PCR [37].

The use of PCR and the methods following PCR for product analysis in diagnostic laboratories requires simplicity, speed, and reproducibility of the methods. More recent 'real time' methods meet these requirements. With the aid of a fluorescence probe, the specific PCR product is detected already while the PCR is being performed by online measurement so that a subsequent product analysis is no longer required. Specific primer/probe sets allow rapid and sensitive detection of influenza viruses in the patient material. A major advantage of this method is the avoidance of contamination since any handling of PCR products becomes unnecessary. Depending on the results to be obtained, primers/probes are used which bind to preserved genome areas, thus permitting the general detection of influenza A and separate detection of influenza B viruses. PCR assays for specific sequence segments are used for differentiation into the various HA and NA subtypes of influenza A viruses [38].

2 Blood and Plasma Donors

The peculiarities listed for the pandemic case refer to Step 6 of the definition of a pandemic according to the WHO (table 1), to the extent that blood donor services are affected. It is therefore necessary for blood donor services to receive the current epidemiological ratings. In the case of a pandemic, an appropriate and co-ordinated reaction of the blood donor services to the current epidemic situation must be made possible by integrating all blood donor services into the pandemic plans of the 'Länder' (German federal states) and laying down the flow of information.

2.1 Prevalence and Incidence in Donor Populations

Reliable data on the prevalence of influenza virus infections in blood donors are not yet available. However, it can be assumed that the prevalence and incidence of the donor collective is comparable with those of the general population.

2.2 Definition of Exclusion Criteria

For influenza virus infections, the general exclusion criteria for febrile infections apply pursuant to the haemotherapy guidelines (Hämotherapie-Richtlinien) [40].

Special Precautions to Be Observed during the Pandemic Period

A risk/benefit analysis could be considered between a breakdown of blood supply and an emergency relaxation of the following donor selection criteria, in close coordination with the competent authorities:

- reduce haemoglobin requirement of 13.5 to 13 g/l for men and from 12.5 to 12 g/l for women (subject to individual decision by the physician),
- increase donation frequency for platelet apheresis,
- increase age limit for multiple donors to approximately 70 years (subject to individual decision by the physician),
- acceptance of donors already 1 week after recovery from influenza if subjective physical well-being has been restored (subject to the decision by the physician),
- influenza prophylaxis using medicinal products is not an exclusion criterion, if no clinical symptoms have appeared.

Table 1. Pandemic phases according to the WHO pandemic preparedness plan [39]

Inter-pandemic period	
Phase 1	No new influenza virus subtypes have been detected in humans. An influenza virus subtype that has caused human infection may be present in animals. If present in animals, the risk of human infection or disease is considered to be low.
Phase 2	No new influenza virus subtypes have been detected in humans. However, a circulating animal influenza virus subtype poses a substantial risk of human disease.
Pandemic alert period	
Phase 3	Human infection(s) with a new subtype, but no human-to-human spread, or at most rare instances of spread to a close contact.
Phase 4	Small cluster(s) with limited human-to-human transmission, but spread is highly localised, suggesting that the virus is not well adapted to humans.
Phase 5	Larger cluster(s) but human-to-human spread still localised, suggesting that the virus is becoming increasingly better adapted to humans, but may not yet be fully transmissible (substantial pandemic risk).
Pandemic period	
Phase 6	Pandemic: increased and sustained transmission in general population. Decisions to be made in Phase 6 whether a country is not yet affected, a country is affected or has close trade relations or travel between an affected country, activity has decreased, or a second pandemic wave has occurred
Post-pandemic phase	
	Return to inter-pandemic period

2.3 Donor Testing and Significance

Donor testing for virus genome of influenza virus is not necessary on the basis of the present data situation.

Special Situation during the Pandemic Period
Donor screening with nucleic acid amplification techniques for the detection of viraemia cannot be introduced immediately from a technical point of view. No validated test systems are available. Up to now, there is no evidence for influenza transmission by blood products. The risk of an infection by blood products compared with the likelihood of infection through social contacts is therefore in all probability negligible. Considering the collection staff shortages to be expected, the use of the additional workload imposed by rapid tests for antigen detection including advice in the event of a positive outcome is questionable compared with the benefit to be expected.

2.4 Donor Interviews

Based on the haemotherapy guidelines (Hämotherapie-Richtlinien) [40], questions to the donor include information on well-being and fever.

Special Situation during the Pandemic Period
Potential donors should be asked expressly whether he/she cared for influenza patients within the past 7 days prior to donation or had comparatively close contacts with influenza-infected individuals.
Admission for donation should be based on these potential donors' current state of health and protective measures they have taken.
The question of general contact with influenza-infected individuals is of little use during a pandemic period.

2.5 Donor Information and Counselling

There is currently no justification for making recommendations regarding donor testing, advice to donors and look-back procedures. Specific donor information takes place.

Special Situation during the Pandemic Period
To prevent masses of people from meeting in one site, special appointments should be made for blood collection activities. Donors should receive MNS masks on entering the donation site and should be offered a hand disinfectant with emphasis. All blood donor services should prepare appropriate information material for blood donors and blood collection staff and train their staff beforehand.

3 Recipients

3.1 Prevalence and Incidence of Blood-Associated Infections and Infectious Diseases in Recipient Populations

No recipient-specific data is available on the prevalence and incidence of influenza virus infections. However, it can be assumed that the prevalence of antibodies against influenza viruses in these collectives is equivalent to that of the general population. No information is available on influenza virus infections transmitted by blood or blood products.

3.2 *Immune Status (Resistance, Existing Immunity, Immune Response, Age, Exogenous Factors)*

Due to the high antigenetic variability of influenza viruses, the continuously emerging drift variants can cause annual influenza epidemics. For this reason, influenza vaccines must be adapted to the current drift variants each year and used in vaccinations to provide highest possible protection. The WHO provides recommendations on the antigen composition of the vaccine before each influenza season. In Germany, according to the Ständige Impfkommission (STIKO; German Standing Vaccination Committee), above all individuals with an increased risk of developing a severe influenza infection (persons over 60 years, patients with underlying disease, chronically ill and immunocompromised persons and persons with an increased risk, such as medical staff) should be immunised yearly. People are protected by the vaccine after 2 weeks. The protection rate is about 70–90% if the vaccine strains coincide well with the circulating strains. Even if the protection rate is clearly lower in the older population, severe disease requiring hospitalisation and fatal outcome is reduced by 50% among the vaccinated population [41, 42].

3.3 *Severity and Course of the Disease*

No reports are available on influenza virus infections by blood products.

3.4 *Therapy and Prophylaxis*

Three antiviral products for the treatment of influenza virus infections are authorised in Germany. Due to adverse reactions, the M2 ion channel blocker amantadine is hardly used. Rimantadine, another member of this class of active ingredients, has fewer side-effects, but is not authorised in Germany. These adamantanes are only effective against influenza A viruses and very rapidly contribute to the development of resistant virus variants [43]. The markedly more effective neuraminidase inhibitors oseltamivir and zanamivir can help shorten the phase of the disease and reduce the symptoms if administered in time (within 24 h after the occurrence of the symptoms if possible) [44]. Nearly all H5N1 isolates from Vietnam and Thailand were adamantine-resistant, whereas most of the H5N1 isolates from Indonesia and China were adamantine-sensitive [45]. The majority of H5N1 viruses from South-East Asia from 2004 were sensitive to the neuraminidase inhibitors oseltamivir and zanamivir. A number of H5N1 isolates were also sensitive to both classes of antiviral substances [19]. Both human and H5N1 viruses may show resistance to oseltamivir, but may be sensitive to zanamivir [46, 47]. Therefore, continued resistance testing should be carried out both for human and for H5N1 strains.

3.5 *Transmissibility*

Influenza is typically transmitted by air or direct contact. Transmissions of human influenza viruses by blood and blood products have so far not been reported, not even during pronounced influenza epidemics. To protect the medical staff in the blood donor services, the decisions on the protection of medical staff adopted by the Ausschuss für biologische Arbeitsstoffe (ABAS, Committee for Biological Substances) should be applied in a way suitable for the situation during an influenza epidemic [48].

3.6 *Frequency of Administration, Type and Amount of Blood Products*

No reports are available so far which show any evidence for a transmission of human influenza viruses by blood products or plasma components.

4 Blood Products

4.1 *Infectious Load of the Starting Material and Test Methods*

The symptoms of an infection with human influenza virus give rise to the assumption that extrapulmonary tissue is infected, which is caused by viraemia. Such a viraemia could be identified several times by isolation of the viruses from the blood. Virus isolation could not only be performed during the symptomatic phase of serious courses of infection [49], but also as early as before the onset of the clinical symptoms during a normal course of the disease [50, 51]. These detections of virus, however, remain limited to isolated cases.
So far, only few data is available on the occurrence of viraemia during an H5N1 infection. However, since severe diarrhoea could be observed in which virus detection was positive, it must be assumed that viraemia can occur with this virus type as well. Such a viraemia is observed in connection with high viral load and fatal outcome [52]. Whether the cases available are isolated cases or whether a general statement can be made remains to be clarified.
In conclusion, it can be stated that viraemia is possible in case of an influenza virus infection, even though the probability is low for the human virus type in case of a normal course of the disease. For H5N1 infections, the situation is judged differently: Based on the prolonged incubation period of up to 7 days

and the apparently more frequent dissemination of the viruses in the blood, the risk potential is rated higher. What remains unclear, however, both for human and for avian influenza viruses, is whether the introduction of virus into the blood circulation will lead to an infection of the blood recipient. In case of a natural infection, the influenza viruses enter the body via the respiratory epithelium where they replicate. So far, available data on the effectiveness of transmission via the blood are not sufficient. This question should be taken into account in future studies.

4.2 Methods for Removal and Inactivation of the Infectious Agent

Influenza viruses belong to the group of enveloped viruses and are, therefore, inactivated by lipid solvents which are also used e.g. in S/D methods. Transmission of influenza viruses by plasma derivatives can therefore be ruled out, above all thanks to the use of physical and chemical depletion and inactivation steps during manufacture [53].

4.3 Feasibility and Validation of Procedures for Removal/ Inactivation of the Infectious Agent

In principle, human influenza isolates can be used for the validation of the manufacturing procedures for plasma components. Since different levels of antibody prevalence against influenza A/H1N1, A/H2N2, and A/H3N2 as well as influenza B viruses are present in the population, this should be taken into account in validating the different methods.

5 Assessment

According to the present state of knowledge, viraemia is observed only in serious courses of infection with human influenza viruses. This viraemia can usually be detected only as late as the first occurrence of symptoms of the disease such as fever. Infections with avian influenza A/H5N1 virus are characterised by the fact that they coincide with a high percentage of severe clinical symptoms and that, in case of fatal outcome, virus can be detected in all organs. It can be assumed that H5N1 infections in humans involve viraemia. Nothing is known about the onset of this viraemic phase following infection. Since the incubation period is 1–7 days for previously observed cases of disease, and is, as a rule, 2–5 days, it can be assumed that the viraemic phase is 7–10 days.

In principle, it can be assumed that plasma components are safe both with regard to human influenza viruses and with regard to avian influenza virus. Special steps during the annual influenza epidemics with human influenza viruses with regard to safety of cellular, non-inactivated blood components are not indicated.

Because of their significance for the guarantee of the population's medical care in the pandemic case, blood donor services would have to be involved in the plans of the competent Federal and 'Länder' Authorities (authorities based on the federal state), and thus in the information flow. Since many of the blood donor services also operate beyond the boundaries of the 'Länder', it is necessary to co-ordinate the efforts between all 'Länder' authorities involved.

For the pandemic case, a framework should also be created enabling the blood donor services to co-ordinate their work as fast as possible. In agreement with the competent 'Länder' authorities, blood donor services will then be able to take steps to guarantee the blood component supply under pandemic conditions too, depending on the current epidemiological situation. Plans have been made to establish an agreement pursuant to section 3 subsection 2 of the Transfusionsgesetz (German Transfusion Act) laying down the details of mutual support in the event of disasters and other emergencies. Such an agreement is currently being compiled by the organisations that run the blood donor services.

This paper was completed on March 19, 2007 and approved by the German Advisory Committee Blood (*Arbeitskreis Blut*) on May 30, 2007. It was compiled by the members of the subgroup 'Assessment of Pathogens Transmissible by Blood' of the German Advisory Committee Blood:

Dr. Johannes Blümel
Prof. Dr. Reinhard Burger
Dr. Christian Drosten
Dr. Albrecht Gröner
Prof. Dr. Lutz Gürtler
Dr. Margarethe Heiden
PD Dr. Martin Hildebrandt
Prof. Dr. Dr. Bernd Jansen
Dr. Horst Klamm
Dr. Thomas Montag-Lessing
Dr. Ruth Offergeld
Prof. Dr. Georg Pauli
Prof. Dr. Rainer Seitz
Dr. Uwe Schlenkrich
Dr. Volkmar Schottstedt
Dr. Hannelore Willkommen
Prof. Dr. Carl-Heinz Wirsing von König
with the special support from Dr. Brunhilde Schweiger (Robert Koch-Institut)

References

1 Wright PF, Webster RG: Orthomyxoviruses; in Fields BN, Knipe DM, Howley PM, et al (eds): Fields Virology, 4th ed. Philadelphia, Lippincott Williams and Wilkins, 2001, pp 1533 ff.

2 Scholtissek C: Stability of infectious influenza A viruses at low pH and at elevated temperature. Vaccine 1985;3(suppl 1):215–218.

3 Fouchier RA, Munster V, Wallensten A, Bestebroer TM, Herfst S, Smith D, Rimmelzwaan GF, Olsen B, Osterhaus AD: Characterization of a novel influenza A virus hemagglutinin subtype (H16) obtained from black-headed gulls. J Virol 2005;79:2814–2822.

4 Rota PA, Wallis TR, Harmon MW, Rota JS, Kendal AP, Nerome K: Cocirculation of two distinct evolutionary lineages of influenza type B virus since 1983. Virology 1990;175:59–68.

5 Nerome R, Hiromoto Y, Sugita S, Tanabe N, Ishida M, Matsumoto M, Lindstrom SE, Takahashi T, Nerome K: Evolutionary characteristics of influenza B virus since its first isolation in 1940: dynamic circulation of deletion and insertion mechanism. Arch Virol 1998;143:1569–1583.

6 Scholtissek C, Rohde W, Von Hoyningen V, Rott R: On the origin of the human influenza virus subtypes H2N2 and H3N2. Virology 1978;87:13–20.

7 Kawaoka Y, Krauss S, Webster RG: Avian-to-human transmission of the PB1 gene of influenza A viruses in the 1957 and 1968 pandemics. J Virol 1989;63:4603–4608.

8 World Health Organization: Avian Influenza. *www.who.int/csr/disease/avian_influenza/en/index.html.*

9 Lyytikäinen O, Hoffmann E, Timm H, Schweiger B, Witte W, Vieth U, Ammon A, Petersen LR: Influenza A outbreak among adolescents in a ski hostel. Eur J Clin Microbiol Infect Dis 1998;17:128–130.

10 Thomas P, Riffelmann M, Schweiger B, Dominik S, von Konig CH: Fatal influenza A virus infection in a child vaccinated against influenza. Pediatr Infect Dis J 2003;22:201–202.

11 Laing R, Slater W, Coles C, Chambers S, Frampton C, Jackson R, Jennings L, Karalus N, Mills G, Murdoch D, Town I: Community-acquired pneumonia in Christchurch and Waikato 1999–2000: microbiology and epidemiology. N Z Med J 2001;114:488–492.

12 Oliveira EC, Marik PE, Colice G: Influenza pneumonia: a descriptive study. Chest 2001;119:1717–1723.

13 de Jong MD, Bach VC, Phan TQ, Vo MH, Tran TT, Nguyen BH, Beld M, Le TP, Truong HK, Nguyen VV, Tran TH, Do QH, Farrar J: Fatal avian influenza A (H5N1) in a child presenting with diarrhea followed by coma. N Engl J Med 2005;352:686–691.

14 Beigel JH, Farrar J, Han AM, Hayden FG, Hyer R, de Jong MD, Lochindarat S, Nguyen TK, Nguyen TH, Tran TH, Nicoll A, Touch S, Yuen KY; Writing Committee of the World Health Organization (WHO) Consultation on human influenza A/H5: Avian influenza A (H5N1) infection in humans. N Engl J Med 2005;353:1374–1385.

15 Yu H, Shu Y, Hu S, Zhang H, Gao Z, Chen H, Dong J, Xu C, Zhang Y, Xiang N, Wang M, Guo Y, Cox N, Lim W, Li D, Wang Y, Yang W: The first confirmed human case of avian influenza A (H5N1) in Mainland China. Lancet 2006;367(9504):84.

16 Webster RG: Influenza: An Emerging Disease. Emerg Infect Dis 1998;4:436–441.

17 Webster RG: The importance of animal influenza for human disease. Vaccine 2002;20(suppl 2):16–20.

18 Gregory V, Bennett M, Orkhan MH, Al Hajjar S, Varsano N, Mendelson E, Zambon M, Ellis J, Hay A, Lin YP: Emergence of influenza A (H1N2) reassortant viruses in the human population during 2001. Virology 2002;300:1–7.

19 Fauci AS: () Seasonal and pandemic influenza preparedness: science and countermeasures. J Infect Dis 2006;194(suppl 2):S73–S76.

20 Zucs P, Buchholz U, Haas W, Uphoff H: Influenza associated excess mortality in Germany, 1985–2001. Emerg Themes Epidemiol 2005;2:6.

21 Arbeitsgemeinschaft Influenza (AGI): Saisonberichte. *www.influenza.rki.de/agi.*

22 Thompson WW, Shay DK, Weintraub E, Brammer L, Cox N, Anderson LJ, Fukuda K: Mortality associated with influenza and respiratory syncytial virus in the United States. JAMA 2003;289:179–186.

23 Schweiger B, Zadow I, Heckler R: Antigenic drift and variability of influenza viruses. Med Microbiol Immunol 2002;191:133–138.

24 Schweiger B: Molecular characterization of human influenza viruses – a look back on the last 10 years. Berl Munch Tierarztl Wochenschr 2006;119:167–178.

25 Schweiger B: Nationale und globale Influenzasurveillance als Basis der jährlichen Impfstoffempfehlung. Bundesgesundheitsbl Gesundheitsforsch Gesundheitsschutz 2001;44:1153–1161.

26 Coonrod JD, Karathanasis P, Betts RF, Donofrio JC: Enzyme-linked immunosorbent assay of core antigens for clinical diagnosis of influenza. J Med Virology 1988;25:399–409.

27 Johnston SLG, Siegel CS: A comparison of direct immunofluorescence, shell vial culture, and conventional cell culture for the rapid detection of influenza A and B. Diagn Microbiol Infect Dis 1991;14: 131–134.

28 Gleaves CA, Brown JA: Detection of influenza A in clinical specimens and cell culture fluid by a commercial EIA. Clin Diagn Virol 1993;1:123–127.

29 Ruest A, Michaud S, Deslandes S, Frost EH: Comparison of the Directigen Flu A+B test, the QuickVue Influenza test, and clinical case definition to viral culture and reverse transcription-PCR for rapid diagnosis of influenza virus infection. J Clin Microbiol 2003;41:3487–3493.

30 Booth S, Baleriola C, Rawlinson WD: Comparison of two rapid influenza A/B test kits with reference methods showing high specificity and sensitivity for influenza A infection. J Med Virol 2006;78:619–622.

31 Donofrio JC, Coonrod JD, Davidson JN, Betts RF: Detection of influenza A and B in respiratory secretions with the polymerase chain reaction. PCR Meth Applicat 1992;1:263–268.

32 Wright KE, Wilson GAR, Novosad D, Dimock C, Tan D, Weber JM: Typing and subtyping of influenza viruses in clinical samples by PCR. J Clin Microbiol 1995;33(5):1180–1184.

33 Claas ECJ, Sprenger MJW, Kleter GEM, van Beek R, Quint WGV, Masurel N: Type-specific identification of influenza viruses A, B and C by the polymerase chain reaction. J Virol Methods 1992;39: 1–13.

34 Yamada A, Imanishi J: Detection of influenza B virus in throat swabs using the polymerase chain reaction. Acta Virol 1992;36:320–325.

35 Schweiger B, Lange I, Heckler R, Willers H, Schreier E: Rapid detection of influenza A neuraminidase subtypes by cDNA amplification coupled to a simple DNA enzyme immunoassay. Arch Virol 1994;139:439–444.

36 Cherian T, Bobo L, Steinhoff MC, Karron RA, Yolken RH: Use of PCR-enzyme immunoassay for identification of influenza A virus matrix RNA in clinical samples negative for cultivable virus. J Clin Microbiol 1994;32:623–628.

37 Zhang WD, Evans DH: Detection and identification of human influenza viruses by the polymerase chain reaction. J Virol Methods 1991;33:165–189.

38 Schweiger B, Zadow I, Heckler R, Timm H, Pauli G: Application of a fluorogenic PCR assay for typing and subtyping of influenza viruses in respiratory samples. J Clin Microbiol 2000;38:1552–1558.

39 WHO Global Influenza Preparedness Plan. The Role of WHO and Recommendations for National Measures before and during Pandemics. WHO/CDS/CSR/GIP/2005.5.

40 Bekanntmachung der Richtlinien zur Gewinnung von Blut und Blutbestandteilen und zur Anwendung von Blutprodukten (Hämotherapie) gemäß §§ 12 und 18 des Transfusionsgesetzes (TFG) (Novelle 2005) vom 19. September 2005. Bundesanzeiger (Sonderheft) Nr. 209a, Jahrgang 57, vom 05.11.2005.

41 Nichol KL: Complications of influenza and benefits of vaccination. Vaccine 1999;17(suppl 1):S47–S52.

42 Vu T, Farish S, Jenkins M, Kelly H: A meta-analysis of effectiveness of influenza vaccine in persons aged 65 years and over living in the community. Vaccine 2002;20:1831–1836.

43 Hayden FG: Antiviral resistance in influenza viruses – implications for management and pandemic response. N Engl J Med 2006;354:785–788.

44 Hayden FG, Pavia AT: Antiviral management of seasonal and pandemic influenza. J Infect Dis 2006; 194(suppl 2):S119–126.

45 Cheung CL, Rayner JM, Smith GJ, Wang P, Naipospos TS, Zhang J, Yuen KY, Webster RG, Peiris JS, Guan Y, Chen H: Distribution of amantadine-resistant H5N1 avian influenza variants in Asia. J Infect Dis 2006;193:1626–1629.

46 Baz M, Abed Y, McDonald J, Boivin G: Characterization of multidrug-resistant influenza A/H3N2 viruses shed during 1 year by an immunocompromised child. Clin Infect Dis 2006;43:1555–1561.

47 Le QM, Kiso M, Someya K, Sakai YT, Nguyen TH, Nguyen KH, Pham ND, Ngyen HH, Yamada S, Muramoto Y, Horimoto T, Takada A, Goto H, Suzuki T, Suzuki Y, Kawaoka Y: Avian flu: isolation of drug-resistant H5N1 virus. Nature 2005;437:1108.

48 Ausschuss für biologische Arbeitsstoffe (ABAS): Arbeitsschutz beim Auftreten von nicht impfpräventabler Influenza unter besonderer Berücksichtigung des Atemschutzes. Beschluss 609. *www.baua.de/nn_15408/de/Themen-von-A-Z/Biologische-Arbeitsstoffe/TRBA/pdf/Beschluss-609.pdf.*

49 Lehmann NI, Gust ID: Viraemia in influenza. A report of two cases. Med J Aust 1971;2:1166–1169.

50 Stanley ED, Jackson GG: Viremia in Asian influenza. Trans Assoc Am Phys 1966;79:376–387.

51 Khakpour M, Saidi A, Naficy K: Proved viraemia in Asian influenza (Hong Kong variant) during incubation period. Br Med J 1969;4:208–209.

52 de Jong MD, Simmons CP, Thanh TT, Hien VM, Smith GJ, Chau TN, Hoang DM, Chau NV, Khanh TH, Dong VC, Qui PT, Cam BV, Ha do Q, Guan Y, Peiris JS, Chinh NT, Hien TT, Farrar J: Fatal outcome of human influenza A (H5N1) is associated with high viral load and hypercytokinemia. Nat Med 2006;12:1203–1207.

53 Kreil TR, Unger U, Orth SM, Petutschnig G, Kistner O, Poelsler G, Berting A: H5N1 influenza virus and the safety of plasma products. Transfusion 2007;47:452–459.

Transfusion Medicine
and Hemotherapy

Transfus Med Hemother 2009;36:40–47
DOI: 10.1159/000197321

Hepatitis E Virus

Arbeitskreis Blut, Untergruppe «Bewertung Blutassoziierter Krankheitserreger»

1 Current Knowledge about the Pathogen

1.1 Characteristics of Hepatitis E

First indications of hepatitis E as a distinct disease, which differs from hepatitis A, were found in 1980 when sensitive and specific detection systems for hepatitis A virus (HAV) first became available and hepatitis epidemics were examined in India. Epidemiologic studies up to that time pointed to the fact that these hepatitis infections with clinically very similar course were caused by HAV pathogens transmitted by the faecal-oral route. The experimental proof that a second virus transmitted by the faecal-oral route, which was later called hepatitis E virus (HEV), was provided in 1983 by the transmission studies of Balayan et al. [1]. In these experiments, HAV-immune voluntary individuals were infected with stool suspensions from patients with a hepatitis A-like disease which occurred in Tashkent, Uzbekistan. Spherical virus-like particles, 27–30 nm in diameter, could be isolated from the stools of the experimentally infected persons, which formed a band in the CsCl gradient at a density of 1.35 g/cm^3. These particles could be detected by immuno-electron microscopy (IEM) both in the pre-clinical (as from the 27th day post infection (dpi)) and in the post-clinical phase (45 dpi, onset of the disease approximately 36 dpi) (fig. 1).

Up to 1990, IEM and the inoculation of monkeys were the only diagnostic methods for the detection of HEV infections and their differentiation from HAV. In 1991, Reyes et al. [2] succeeded in cloning the genome. This opened new paths for the development of diagnostic methods for serological and molecular detection of HEV infections. HEV was first categorised as part of the Caliciviridae family, based on its morphological properties. Sequence analysis, however, revealed that the genome structure of HEV is significantly distinct from this virus family. Therefore, HEV is today classified as the so far only representative of the hepevirus genus in the new family of Hepeviridae.

HEV is a small non-enveloped, single-stranded icosaedric virus with a diameter of approximately 32–34 nm. The capsid of the virus probably consists of one single protein. The genome is single-stranded positive-sense with a size of 7.2 kbp. It is flanked by non-encoding regions, polyadenylated at the 3' end, and bears a m^{7}G-cap at the 5' end. The genome itself encodes for three overlapping open reading frames (ORF 1–3). Hepeviruses have the feature that the ORF 2 with a length of 2 kbp located at the 3' end encodes for the capsid protein. It is especially this characteristic that makes the HEV virus distinct from the calicivirus, in which the sequence encoding for the capsid is located at the 5' end. ORF 1 with a length of approximately 5 kbp is located at the 5' end and encodes for the non-structural proteins involved in RNA replication: RNA-dependent RNA polymerase, guanylyl and methyl transferases, helicase and a papain-like protease. ORF 3 with a length of 372 bp overlaps at the 3' end with the first 331 bp from ORF 2 and at the 5' end with ORF 1. ORF 3 encodes for a small immunogeneic phosphoprotein with a size of not more than 123 amino acids.

Based on phylogenetic analyses, the isolates examined up to now are classified into four different genotypes which have different world-wide distributions [3]. For genotype 1 the Burma isolate represents the prototype, for genotype 2 the Mexican isolate, for genotype 3 the USA isolate, and for genotype 4 the Chinese isolate. The different genotypes are then further grouped into different genetic subtypes. Serologically, HEV seems to behave in a uniform manner, as neutralisation studies in the cell culture and protection studies with different genotypes in infection studies have shown [4].

Various studies provide evidence that HEV replicates in hepatocyte culture of humans and macaques. For this purpose, cell cultures were infected with HEV from stool suspensions. In such in vitro studies, Emerson et al. [5] were able to show that approximately half the HEV infectiveness was inactivated after heat treatment at 45–50 °C for 1 h and almost the entire HEV infectiveness at 56 °C. In addition, the authors were able

KARGER

Fax +49 761 4 52 07 14
Information@Karger.de
www.karger.com

Accessible online at:
www.karger.com/tmh

Previously published in Transfus Med Hemother 2008;35:50–57

to show that, although different HEV isolates showed different degrees of heat stability, all isolates studied were sensitive to treatment at 60 °C for 1 h. In contrast to this, only half of the HAV could be inactivated when treated at 60 °C for 1 h and lost its infectiveness only after heat treatment at 66 °C. These findings thus revealed that HEV was more sensitive to heat than HAV [5]. Tanaka et al. [6] completed the thermostability studies of HEV with cell culture-adapted HEV. Heat treatment of HEV at 90 °C for 1 min or at 70 °C for 10 min inactivated HEV entirely. Incubation of HEV suspensions at 56 °C for 30 min reduced the titre in comparison to treatment at 25 °C.

1.2 Infection and Infectious Diseases

The course of HEV infections is similar to that of HAV infections. As a rule, acute HEV infection is self-limiting with a low death rate, which is, however, higher (0.5–4%) than that of the HAV infection (approximately 0.2%) [7]. HEV is usually transmitted by the faecal-oral route and is excreted in the stool for 3–4 weeks. In some patients, an excretion period of up to 120 days could be observed using PCR [8]. It is assumed that HEV first replicates in the intestinal duct and then reaches the liver via the blood vessels. There, replication of the virus takes place in the cytoplasm of hepatocytes. The virus is then excreted into the stool and the blood via the gall. The incubation period measured by the increase in transaminases can be between 3 and 8 weeks. In the acute incubation phase up to the late phase, the virus is excreted via the stool in high quantities [1]. Experimental oral infections of humans showed that viraemia was first detectable between the 22nd and the 28th dpi, approximately 1 week before the occurrence of symptoms [1, 9]. Symptoms of the disease then occurred between the 30th and the 36th dpi. The peak of the transaminases was observed at approximately the same time as the appearance of the first antibodies. Histologically, focal necroses and apoptosis of cells are found in the liver. Whether the observed alterations are caused by the virus itself or by the immune response is unclear, since only minor signs of inflammation could be detected [10]. Comparable courses of infection were also observed in experimental transmissions of HEV to primates [11, 12].

Similarly to hepatitis A, an IgM and an IgG response can be measured at approximately the time of the occurrence of symptoms in the acute HEV infection.

HEV infections during pregnancy have a high percentage of serious outcomes, accompanied by a high mortality rate of approximately 20%. The mortality rate in men and non-pregnant women is 0.5–4% [7, 10, 13, 14]. In addition to the serious liver failure which is observed in particular in pregnant women in their third trimester, encephalopathies and disseminated intravascular consumptive coagulation disorders can occur.

In the past few years, there have been an increasing number of reports about HEV infections with sub-clinical course [15, 16]. Increased levels of transaminases may act as infection markers. In this phase, HEV genome is detectable in the blood in a high percentage of the infected individuals. More or less simultaneously, an increase in the HEV-specific IgM and IgG antibody responses are observed. Transmissions of HEV by non-inactivated blood products from such donors have been reported from various countries [17–21].

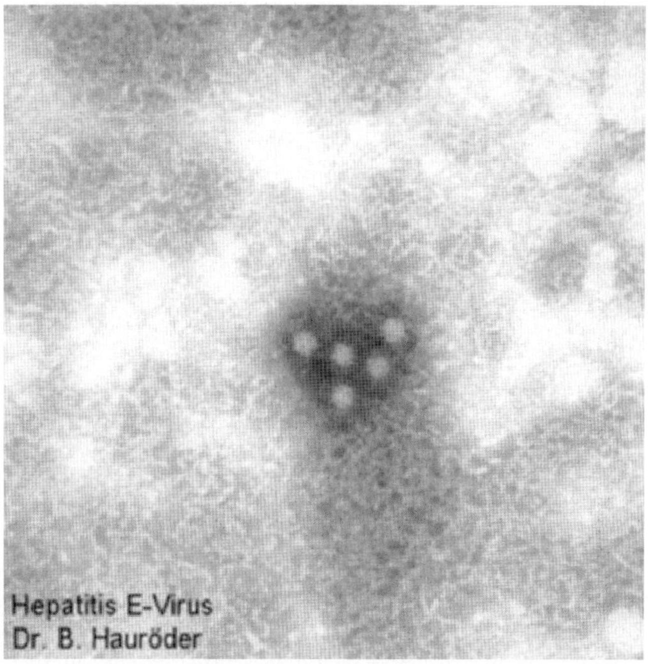

Fig. 1. Electron microscope photo of an immune aggregate of HEV isolated from the gall of an experimentally infected macaques. The infectious HEV was isolated from the faeces of an individual with HEV. The monkeys were infected orally. We thank Dr. Bärbel Hauröder, *Zentrales Institut des Sanitätsdienstes der Bundeswehr Koblenz* (Central Institute of the Paramedic Services of the *Bundeswehr* (German army) at Koblenz, Germany).

1.3 Epidemiology

Acute hepatitis E is a very frequent cause of hepatitis acquired by the faecal-oral route world-wide. For a long time, HEV, the causative agent of this disease, was considered as a human-specific pathogen. As far as geographic distribution is concerned, one distinguishes between those regions, where HEV occurs endemically, and those where it is sporadic [22]. In this context, Southeast and Central Asia, the Middle East, Africa and Central America are considered as endemic areas. In these regions, pronounced epidemics have been observed in the past few decades, which were frequently caused by contaminated drinking water, but isolated sporadic cases of HEV infection have also been reported.

Table 1. Notifications of HEV infections in compliance with the IfSG (Infection Protection Act) (Source: Robert Koch-Institut)

Year	Cases of HEV reported in Germany	
	total	acquired in Germany
2001	31	11
2002	17	7
2003	33	10
2004	53	21
2005	54	23
2006	51	23

In the industrialised countries of Europe and America, HEV infections as a rule only occurred in travellers who had previously stayed in endemic areas. In the past few years, however, more and more reports have been published stating that sporadic hepatitis E also occurs in non-endemic areas, i.e. industrialised countries, without any connection with travelling to classic endemic areas [23, 24].

Most of the serious HEV infections in Asia and Africa are caused by genotype 1 while genotype 2 predominates in Mexico, Egypt, Nigeria, and Namibia. Genotype 3 has been observed in Asia, America and Europe as well as in New Zealand. The recently newly described genotype 4 has up to now been observed mainly in Asia [3, 25]. According to findings established, genotypes 1 and 2 have mainly been found with disease in humans in the respective endemic areas. Genotypes 3 and 4, however, have been found both in humans and in animals, especially domestic and wild pigs [25].

Animals, especially pigs, are regarded as the source of the infectious pathogens for humans in industrialised countries. Hepatitis E is therefore to an increasing extent considered to be a zoonosis. HEV was first detected successfully in a pig in the USA in 1997 [26]. A high HEV prevalence rate is shown in pigs in nearly all regions of the world [22]. Evidence for this could be provided by serological, virological and molecular detection methods. In addition, the close relationship of isolates from humans and pigs in the respective regions could be shown by phylogenetic analyses of the virus genomes.

Experimental infections in primates and pigs with HEV, and in pigs with human isolates, support the hypothesis that hepatitis E is a zoonosis [27]. Apart from pigs, HEV was detected in various other species such as rats, dogs and birds. It has so far been unclear which role these species play in the transmission to humans.

Sporadic outbreaks of HEV infection in Japan were attributed to the consumption of insufficiently cooked or raw pork, venison or boar meat [28]. This assumption has been supported by studies performed by Feagins et al. [29] who were able to isolate infectious HEV from commercial pork liver in the USA.

Studies on the prevalence of HEV infections both in humans and in pigs were performed in various European countries. Studies in Spain have shown that HEV is very widespread in pig populations and that an age-dependent increase in the seroprevalence can be observed [30]. Furthermore, HEV could be detected in the faeces of the animals by NAT/PCR in the age group of 8–12 weeks. Comparable results were also obtained when studying pig populations in the Netherlands, where HEV genome could be detected in the faeces in a high percentage of the fattening farms [31]. A close relationship between human and porcine HEV was reported from the UK [32, 33].

Altogether, only few studies are available on the prevalence of HEV infections in humans. High antibody prevalence with approximately 13% has been reported from Sweden and lower antibody prevalence from France and Spain (approximately 3%) [34, 35]. In various studies, persons with close contact to pigs such as pig breeders and animal traders showed a higher seroprevalence compared with the general population [36, 37]. This indicates that pigs can be regarded as one of the transmitters of HEV to humans.

Tests of urban sewage water in various industrialised countries showed that for example in Barcelona (Spain), Nancy (France), and Washington, DC (USA) HEV genome could be detected, pointing to the fact that HEV infections in these countries may frequently take a subclinical course and remain undetected, since no simultaneous clinical HEV infection were observed [38]. The extent to which HEV is transmitted by insufficiently purified sewage water in industrialised countries remains unclear.

Only little information is available on the prevalence and incidence of HEV infections in Germany. It has been discussed for a long time whether acute hepatitis E only occurs in travellers returning from endemic areas [39]. More recent studies have revealed that HEV infections can also be acquired in Germany, and can lead to acute courses of disease [40, 41]. Data obtained on the basis of the requirement to notify hepatitis infections in compliance with the IfSG (Infektionsschutzgesetz; Infection Protection Act) show that approximately half of the German hepatitis E cases notified were acquired in Germany, and that there was no connection with travels to endemic areas (table 1). The few HEV cases which have so far been phylogenetically analysed in Germany confirm the close relationship to pig isolates found in various other European countries [41].

1.4 Detection Methods and Their Significance

Up to now it has not been possible to grow HEV routinely in cell culture for diagnostic purposes. Before molecular detection methods were established, virus detection was performed in the faeces by means of electron microscopy or IEM.

Today, HEV can be reliably detected using PCR in the acute phase from faeces or blood. The nucleic acid detection method and sequence analyses of the amplificates, however, have shown that there is a great number of genetic HEV variants. The sensitivity of the PCR therefore depends on the homology of the primer with the isolate to be examined. The extent to

which real-time PCR and nested PCR systems are suitable for the detection of all 4 genotypes known up to now requires further examination [42–44]. Detection of viral RNA confirms the presence of active HEV.
The extent to which antigen detection systems are suitable for the detection of viraemia can only be clarified by further development of experimental antigen detection systems [45].
Serological detection systems for diagnosing an HEV infection still represent the method of choice. Commercial antibody detection systems (ELISA) are available for the detection of IgG and/or IgM antibodies. These systems are based on recombinant ORF 2 and ORF 3 proteins expressed or synthetic peptides. Immunoblots based on recombinant proteins can be used for confirming the reactive sera.
At the time of first detection of HEV antibodies and the presence of clear clinical symptoms of hepatitis, an HEV infection is likely, if hepatitis A, B and C can be excluded. To confirm, a second sample should be drawn 8–10 days later, in order to provide evidence for the increase in antibodies. In approximately 90% of the acute HEV infections, IgM antibodies can be detected 1–4 weeks after occurrence of the clinical symptoms. As a rule, these IgM antibodies can no longer be detected 3 months after the onset of the disease. More recent findings show, however, that anti-HEV IgA antibodies may provide a reliable way of detecting an acute HEV infection [24, 46].
The postulation that a stay in an endemic area of HEV should be one of the criteria for a suspected hepatitis E diagnosis can no longer be maintained based on the current state of knowledge. Studies on the spread of HEV in non-epidemic areas give rise to the assumption that HEV infections may take on an asymptomatic or subclinical course in industrialised countries.

2 Blood and Plasma Donors

2.1 Prevalence and Incidence in Donor Populations

Data on the prevalence of HEV infections in blood and plasma donors and/or in the general population are not available in Germany. In Japan, a country in which only sporadic cases of HEV have been reported, studies have been performed in 6,700 blood donors with elevated transaminases [16]. HEV-specific antibodies could be determined in 7.1% of the individuals studied. In 9 (0.13% of the samples studied) of these blood donors, HEV RNA could be detected, with 6 of these donors also showing anti-HEV IgM and/or IgA antibodies. Three donors were only HEV genome-positive. The authors rule out that in Japan, a country with a comparatively low number of reported acute HEV infections, more subclinical cases occur than expected. It must, however, be assumed that the prevalence in the donor cohort is comparable with that of the overall population. These results confirm previous reports from Japan that HEV was detected in blood donors by means of PCR [47]. To what extent antigen detection systems are suitable for detecting viraemia can only be clarified by the further development of experimental antigen detection systems [45]. Studies of blood donors in HEV-endemic areas such as India give rise to the assumption that in such countries there is an increased risk of transfusion-transmitted HEV [48].
Investigations performed on small random samples of blood donors in the Netherlands showed that 0.4% of the donations were HEV antibody-positive [49], while the number in Spain was 2.8% of the donations tested [34]. In France, a prevalence of 3.2% was determined in blood donors, with only 20–30 autochthonous cases reported annually in that country [35].
In a multi-centre study in 1993, data were collected on the prevalence of HEV infections in Germany [50]. In this study the prevalence of 0.5% HEV antibody-positive donors determined is possibly too low, since the sensitivity of the tests has meanwhile been improved. The number of autochthonous hepatitis E cases reported for Germany is comparable with that of France so that it cannot be ruled out that HEV seroprevalence in Germany is similar to that in France.

2.2 Definition of Exclusion Criteria

The guidelines of the Bundesärztekammer (German Medical Association) and the Paul-Ehrlich-Institut (PEI) [51, 52] form the basis for the exclusion criteria for blood donors. Individuals who are or have been diseased with infectious hepatitis of unclear aetiology should be permanently deferred from donating blood. These guidelines, however, do not deal explicitly with HEV infection. In the event of confirmed or suspected hepatitis E, the donors must be deferred from the donation. This also applies to suspected acute infection of persons who are in a close contact with the donor. Status after overcoming hepatitis E, or determination of anti-HEV IgG antibody confirming recovery from hepatitis E, is not an exclusion criterion. This recommendation is equivalent to the procedure for individuals who recovered from HAV infection [53].

2.3 Donor Testing and Significance

Donor testing for HEV genome by means of PCR or antibody detection (IgM and/or IgA as early infection markers) is possible in principle. Based on the findings available up to now on the epidemiology of HEV infections in Germany, donor testing for virus genome of HEV or HEV-specific antibodies is not considered necessary.

2.4 Donor Interviews

The volunteer who intends to donate blood is asked whether he/she has had a history of hepatitis before each donation, in accordance with the guidelines of the Bundesärztekammer and the PEI. Recovery from a hepatitis E infection in the history is not a criterion for a general donor deferral.

2.5 Donor Information and Counselling

Since no special examination for HEV markers is performed, no HEV-specific donor information is necessary. If there are signs of hepatitis infection of unclear origin, HEV can be detected by using serological or molecular methods.

3 Recipients

3.1 Prevalence and Incidence of Blood-Associated Infections and Infectious Diseases in Recipient Populations

Neither donor- nor recipient-specific information is available on the prevalence and incidence of HEV infections in Germany. It can, however, be assumed that there is a prevalence for antibodies against HEV in these collectives which corresponds to that of the general population, as also described for other European countries.
Studies, in particular in Japan, give rise to the assumption that transmissions of HEV by blood transfusion can be observed. Retrospective data collections, particularly in transfusion recipients displaying increased transaminase values or a serious hepatitis infection, showed that part of these patients had acquired an HEV infection due to this transfusion [19, 34, 48].
Recently, HEV transmissions by transfusion have also been reported from Europe [20, 21]. Haemodialysis patients seem to have an increased infection risk [54]. To what extent this is due to the administration of blood products or has a different cause is unclear. Only few studies on haemophiliacs have been described in the literature [49, 55, 56]; none of these studies pointed to a recognisable transmission risk for HEV by coagulation factors.

3.2 Immune Status (Resistance, Existing Immunity, Immune Response, Age, Exogenous Factors)

No results are available on the prevalence rate among the recipients of blood and blood products in Germany.

3.3 Severity and Course of the Disease

Reports on HEV infections by contaminated blood products give rise to the assumption that the course of infection is comparable to that of a natural HEV infection [19]. Persisting infection following transfusion was reported in a T-lymphoma patient who was also receiving chemotherapy [57].

3.4 Therapy and Prophylaxis

Studies on possible passive immunisation have been reported [58], and the administration of anti-HEV immunoglobulin products as post-exposure prevention, especially for pregnant women, has been discussed.
The development of a vaccine has so far been hampered because HEV has been difficult to replicate in cell culture and because vaccines on the basis of inactivated viruses or non-pathogenic isolates have therefore not been available. The focus of vaccine development was therefore on DNA technology or recombinant proteins [59–63]. One candidate for a DNA vaccine is currently undergoing phase II of a clinical study [63].

3.5 Transmissibility

Retrospective studies by Arankalle and Chobe [17, 48] give reason to presume that HEV can be transmitted by blood transfusions in regions where it is endemic. Transfusion-associated HEV transmissions were reported from Saudi-Arabia, a country where HEV occurs endemically [18]. First reports on transfusion-associated HEV infections from Japan, which has not been rated as an endemic region, were published almost simultaneously [19, 54]. In one case, it could be demonstrated that transmission occurred by transfusion of FFP, but not by the corresponding red blood cell concentrate from the same donor [19].
A case of transfusion-associated HEV transmission has recently been reported also in Europe in a region in which acute hepatitis E occurs only sporadically. In the UK, a patient was infected by a red blood cell concentrate. This concentrate only contained small amounts of plasma from the donor. Another patient who had received a platelet concentrate from the same donation was not infected [20]. A child in France was also infected by a red blood cell concentrate [21]. Both the donor in the UK and the donor in France had acquired their HEV infection in their own countries. Both blood donors were HEV RNA-positive at the time of the donation but did not show elevated transaminases.
As can be concluded from the few more exactly scrutinised HEV transmission cases, HEV can be transmitted by non-inactivated blood components. It can be assumed that this is the case especially during the viraemia phase (approximately 20–50 days following infection) by cell-free virus in the plasma.

3.6 Frequency of Administration, Type and Amount of Blood Products

No conclusions can be drawn from the few reported cases of transmission as to an increased risk of an HEV infection by frequent treatment with non-inactivated blood components, even though several of the patients affected received transfusions from multiple sources.

4 Blood Products

4.1 Infectious Load of the Starting Material and Test Methods

Up to now, no tests have been performed on the viral HEV burden of the starting material. In principle, such a test on these materials for HEV genome would be possible by means of NAT.

4.2 Methods for Removal and Inactivation of the Infectious Agent

There are no investigations on the removal and inactivation of HEV in blood products. In the past few years, animal caliciviruses such as the feline calicivirus (FeCV) were used as model viruses for the validation of inactivation methods. To what extent these model systems reflect the stability of HEV is unclear.

4.3 Feasibility and Validation of Procedures for Removal/Inactivation of the Infectious Agent

In general, procedures of inactivation and/or removal of non-enveloped viruses during the preparation of plasma products are more limited than those for enveloped viruses. The assessment of the capacity of methods of inactivating and/or removing HEV is currently based on the experience with non-enveloped model viruses from other virus groups, especially from FeCV. Studies with HEV itself are available only to a very limited extent, since culturing adapted HEV isolates is difficult, and the cell culture systems are available to only a limited extent. Whether these systems are suitable for validating production steps during the manufacture of blood products remains to be examined.

In the past few years, studies on the thermostability of HEV were carried out. Compared with HAV, HEV proved to be less thermostable [5]. However, in these studies, no exact kinetics of inactivation was displayed, and no stabilisers applied in the production of coagulation factors were investigated.

Preliminary studies show an effective inactivation of FeCV at 60 °C in liquid phase in the presence of such stabilisers (Blümel et al., unpublished; Gröner et al., unpublished). However, to what extent FeCV reflects the heat stability of HEV is unknown. The stability of FeCV and HEV during dry heat application is also unknown.

Stability at low pH values (pH 3.7–4.2) as it is used in the production of antibody preparations is also unknown. Extrapolation from the inactivation data from other non-enveloped viruses is difficult. HAV and animal parvoviruses are usually stable under these conditions.

It can be assumed that filtration methods (virus filter, nanofilter) remove HEV effectively from the product if filters were used which remove smaller viruses such as HAV or parvoviruses. Such filters are often used in the production of factor IX or partly in the production of immunoglobulin preparations. For the filtration of complex coagulation factors, however, only filters with medium diameters of 35–50 nm are often used. In this case the retention of HEV or calicivirus is limited and may strongly depend on specific filters or production conditions. This should be evaluated on a case-to-case basis.

The risk of an HEV transmission by plasma products is currently estimated to be low since steps have been introduced for most of the products (except for SD-treated plasma) which are considered to be at least partly effective in activating or removing HEV. A more accurate assessment of the risk, however, is currently not possible since important data on the epidemiology, the HEV burden in the plasma pool, the prevalence of antibodies in plasma donations and/or plasma pools, and on the inactivation/removal of HEV during the manufacturing process is not available. A product-specific examination of the manufacturing procedures for inactivation/removal of HEV is required in those cases in which the data available on non-enveloped model viruses cannot clearly be transferred to HEV.

The effectiveness of the inactivation methods developed for plasma and cellular blood products (treatment with amotosalen, riboflavin, or methylene blue) is currently unknown. A risk of HEV transmission by blood components can therefore currently not be ruled out in general.

5 Assessment

For a long time, hepatitis E was considered as travel-associated disease. Today, however, evidence has been found that HEV infections not only occur in classical endemic areas with a low standard of hygiene but also in industrialised countries. In the classical endemic areas, particularly the HEV genotypes 1 and 2 have been found. The pathogen is transmitted by the faecal-oral route via contaminated water and food. In non-endemic areas, mainly sporadic HEV infections of the genotypes 3 and 4 are observed. Animals, mainly pigs, provide the reservoir for these two genotypes. Based on the current state of knowledge, pig populations world-wide show a very high HEV infection rate. Phylogenetically closely related viruses are found in industrialised countries in humans with HEV infections and in pigs. Although only low numbers of autochthonous human HEV infections have been reported in industrialised countries, the seroprevalence is relatively high, reaching approximately 13%, e.g. in Sweden.

These findings give rise to the assumption that a considerable number of HEV infections in industrialised countries shows a subclinical course, and that these infections can only be detected by the identification of the HEV genome and/or seroconversion. It has been shown that not only individuals during the incubation and the clinical phase of hepatitis E, but also subclinically infected individuals display HEV viraemia, and that the virus can also be transmitted by blood donations from such donors.

The risk of HEV transmission by blood products has not been sufficiently examined in Germany. Data are missing on the prevalence of HEV infections in the population, in the blood donor collective, and in individuals with a higher risk of exposure for HEV such as veterinarians, pig breeders, pig fatteners, and the staff of abattoirs and butcher businesses. Moreover, there is no information on the prevalence and incidence of HEV in the animal reservoir for Germany, particularly in pig populations. The current state of knowledge is not sufficient to judge the necessity of blood donor testing for HEV genome or HEV antibodies. Based on clinical experience, these tests do not seem to be necessary considering the current epidemiological situation. However, there is a major need for research, especially for collecting epidemiological data, and with regard to targeted look-back tests for transfusion-associated HEV infection in transfusion recipients and the corresponding donors.

This paper was completed on June 22, 2007, and approved by the German Advisory Committee Blood (Arbeitskreis Blut) on October 1, 2007. It was compiled by the members of the subgroup 'Assessment of Pathogens Transmissible by Blood' of the German Advisory Committee Blood (Arbeitskreis Blut):

Prof. Dr. Georg Pauli
Dr. Johannes Blümel
Prof. Dr. Reinhard Burger
Prof. Dr. Christian Drosten
Dr. Albrecht Gröner
Prof. Dr. Lutz Gürtler
Dr. Margarethe Heiden
PD Dr. Martin Hildebrandt
Prof. Dr. Dr. Bernd Jansen
Dr. Horst Klamm
Dr. Thomas Montag-Lessing
Dr. Ruth Offergeld
Prof. Dr. Rainer Seitz
Dr. Uwe Schlenkrich
Dr. Volkmar Schottstedt
Dr. Hannelore Willkommen
Prof. Dr. Carl-Heinz Wirsing von König

References

1 Balayan MS, Andjaparidze AG, Savinskaya SS, Ketiladze ES, Braginsky DM, Savinov AP, Poleschuk VF: Evidence for a virus in non-A, non-B hepatitis transmitted via the fecal-oral route. Intervirology 1983;20:23–31.
2 Reyes GR, Yarbough PO, Tam AW, Purdy MA, Huang CC, Kim JS, Bradley DW, Fry KE: Hepatitis E virus (HEV): the novel agent responsible for enterically transmitted non-A, non-B hepatitis. Gastroenterol Jpn 1991;26(suppl 3):142–147.
3 Lu L, Li C, Hagedorn CH: Phylogenetic analysis of global hepatitis E virus sequences. Genetic diversity, subtypes and zoonosis. Rev Med Virol 2006;16: 5–36.
4 Emerson SU, Purcell RH: Recombinant vaccines for hepatitis E. Trends Mol Med 2001;7:462–466.
5 Emerson SU, Arankalle VA, Purcell RH: Thermal stability of hepatitis E virus. J Infect Dis 2005;192: 930–933.
6 Tanaka T, Takahashi M, Kusano E, Okamoto H: Development and evaluation of an efficient cell-culture system for hepatitis E virus. J Gen Virol 2007;88:903–911.
7 Previsani N, Lavanchy D: Hepatitis E – WHO/CDS/CRS/EDC/2001.12. Geneva: World Health Organisation, Department of Communicable Disease Surveillance and Response, 2001. *www.who.int/csr/disease/hepatitis/HepatitisE_whocdscsredc2001_12.pdf*.
8 Nanda SK, Ansari IH, Acharya SK, Jameel S, Panda SK: Protracted viremia during acute sporadic hepatitis E virus infection. Gastroenterology 1995;108:225–230.
9 Chauhan A, Jameel S, Dilawari JB, Chawla YK, Kaur U, Ganguly NK: Hepatitis E virus transmission to a volunteer. Lancet 1993;341:149–150.
10 Emerson SU, Purcell RH: Hepatitis E virus; in Knipe DM, et al. (eds): Fields Virology, 5th ed. Philadelphia, Lippincott Williams and Wilkins, 2007, p 78.
11 Purcell RH, Emerson SU: Animal models of hepatitis A and E. ILAR J 2001;42:161–177.
12 Zhang J, Ge SX, Huang GY, Li SW, He ZQ, Wang YB, Zheng YJ, Gu Y, Ng MH, Xia NS: Evaluation of antibody-based and nucleic acid-based assays for diagnosis of hepatitis E virus infection in a rhesus monkey model. J Med Virol 2003;71:518–526.
13 Hussaini SH, Skidmore SJ, Richardson P, Sherratt LM, Cooper BT, O'Grady JG: Severe hepatitis E infection during pregnancy. J Viral Hepat 1997;4: 51–54.
14 Jilani N, Das BC, Husain SA, Baweja UK, Chattopadhya D, Gupta RK, Sardana S, Kar P: Hepatitis E virus infection and fulminant hepatic failure during pregnancy. J Gastroenterol Hepatol 2007;22: 676–682.
15 Mitsui T, Tsukamoto Y, Suzuki S, Yamazaki C, Masuko K, Tsuda F, Takahashi M, Tsatsralt-Od B, Nishizawa T, Okamoto H: Serological and molecular studies on subclinical hepatitis E virus infection using periodic serum samples obtained from healthy individuals. J Med Virol 2005;76:526–533.
16 Gotanda Y, Iwata A, Ohnuma H, Yoshikawa A, Mizoguchi H, Endo K, Takahashi M, Okamoto H: Ongoing subclinical infection of hepatitis E virus among blood donors with an elevated alanine aminotransferase level in Japan. J Med Virol 2007; 79:734–742.
17 Arankalle VA, Chobe LP: Retrospective analysis of blood transfusion recipients: evidence for post-transfusion hepatitis E. Vox Sang 2000;79:72–74.
18 Khuroo MS, Kamili S, Yattoo GN: Hepatitis E virus infection may be transmitted through blood transfusions in an endemic area. J Gastroenterol Hepatol 2004;19:778–784.
19 Matsubayashi K, Nagaoka Y, Sakata H, Sato S, Fukai K, Kato T, Takahashi K, Mishiro S, Imai M, Takeda N, Ikeda H: Transfusion-transmitted hepatitis E caused by apparently indigenous hepatitis E virus strain in Hokkaido, Japan. Transfusion 2004; 44:934–940.
20 Boxall E, Herborn A, Kochethu G, Pratt G, Adams D, Ijaz S, Teo CG: Transfusion-transmitted hepatitis E in a 'nonhyperendemic' country. Transfus Med 2006;16:79–83.
21 Colson P, Coze C, Gallian P, Henry M, De Micco P, Tamalet C: Transfusion-associated hepatitis E, France. Emerg Infect Dis 2007;13:648–649.
22 Meng XJ, Dea S, Engle RE, Friendship R, Lyoo YS, Sirinarumitr T, Urairong K, Wang D, Wong D, Yoo D, Zhang Y, Purcell RH, Emerson SU: Prevalence of antibodies to the hepatitis E virus in pigs from countries where hepatitis E is common or is rare in the human population. J Med Virol 1999;59: 297–302.
23 Peron JM, Mansuy JM, Izopet J, Vinel JP: Hepatitis E virus: An emerging disease. Sante 2006;16: 239–243.
24 Herremans M, Duizer E, Jusic E, Koopmans MP: Detection of hepatitis E virus-specific immunoglobulin A in patients infected with hepatitis E virus genotype 1 or 3. Clin Vaccine Immunol 2007; 14:276–280.
25 Okamoto H: Genetic variability and evolution of hepatitis E virus. Virus Res 2007;127:216–228.
26 Meng XJ, Purcell RH, Halbur PG, Lehman JR, Webb DM, Tsareva TS, Haynes JS, Thacker BJ, Emerson SU: A novel virus in swine is closely related to the human hepatitis E virus. Proc Natl Acad Sci U S A 1997;94:9860–9865.
27 Meng XJ: Novel strains of hepatitis E virus identified from humans and other animal species: is hepatitis E a zoonosis? J Hepatol 2000;33:842–845.

28 Matsuda H, Okada K, Takahashi K, Mishiro S: Severe hepatitis E virus infection after ingestion of uncooked liver from a wild boar. J Infect Dis 2003; 188:944.
29 Feagins AR, Opriessnig T, Guenette DK, Halbur PG, Meng XJ: Detection and characterization of infectious hepatitis E virus from commercial pig livers sold in local grocery stores in the USA. J Gen Virol 2007;88:912–917.
30 Seminati C, Mateu E, Peralta B, de Deus N, Martin M: Distribution of hepatitis E virus infection and its prevalence in pigs on commercial farms in Spain. Vet J 2007:DOI 10.1016/j.tvjl.2006.11.018.
31 Rutjes SA, Lodder WJ, Bouwknegt M, de Roda Husman AM: Increased hepatitis E virus prevalence on Dutch pig farms from 33 to 55% by using appropriate internal quality controls for RT-PCR. J Virol Methods 2007;143:112–116.
32 Banks M, Bendall R, Grierson S, Heath G, Mitchell J, Dalton H: Human and porcine hepatitis E virus strains, United Kingdom. Emerg Infect Dis 2004;10: 953–955.
33 Dalton HR, Thurairajah PH, Fellows HJ, Hussaini HS, Mitchell J, Bendall R, Banks M, Ijaz S, Teo CG, Levine DF: Autochthonous hepatitis E in southwest England. J Viral Hepat 2007;14:304–309.
34 Mateos ML, Camarero C, Lasa E, Teruel JL, Mir N, Baquero F: Hepatitis E virus: relevance in blood donors and risk groups. Vox Sang 1999;76:78–80.
35 Boutrouille A, Bakkali-Kassimi L, Cruciere C, Pavio N: Prevalence of anti-hepatitis E virus antibodies in French blood donors. J Clin Microbiol 2007;45:2009–2010.
36 Meng XJ, Wiseman B, Elvinger F, Guenette DK, Toth TE, Engle RE, Emerson SU, Purcell RH: Prevalence of antibodies to hepatitis E virus in veterinarians working with swine and in normal blood donors in the United States and other countries. J Clin Microbiol 2002;40:117–122.
37 Olsen B, Axelsson-Olsson D, Thelin A, Weiland O: Unexpected high prevalence of IgG-antibodies to hepatitis E virus in Swedish pig farmers and controls. Scand J Infect Dis 2006;38:55–58.
38 Clemente-Casares P, Pina S, Buti M, Jardi R, Martin M, Bofill-Mas S, Girones R: Hepatitis E virus epidemiology in industrialized countries. Emerg Infect Dis 2003;9:448–454.
39 Trautwein C, Kiral G, Tillmann HL, Witteler H, Michel G, Manns MP: Risk factors and prevalence of hepatitis E in German immigrants from the former Soviet Union. J Med Virol 1995;45:429–434.
40 Teich N, Tannapfel A, Ammon A, Ruf BR, van der Poe WHM, Mössner J, Liebert UG: Sporadic acute hepatitis E in Germany: an underdiagnosed phenomenon? Z Gastroenterol 2003;41:419–423.
41 Preiss JC, Plentz A, Engelmann E, Schneider T, Jilg W, Zeitz M, Duchmann R: Autochthonous hepatitis E virus infection in Germany with sequence similarities to other European isolates. Infection 2006; 34:173–175.
42 Ahn J, Rayamajhi N, Gyun Kang S, Sang Yoo H: Comparison of real-time reverse transcriptase–polymerase chain reaction and nested or commercial reverse transcriptase–polymerase chain reaction for the detection of hepatitis E virus particle in human serum. Diagn Microbiol Infect Dis 2006; 56:269–274.
43 Enouf V, Dos Reis G, Guthmann JP, Guerin PJ, Caron M, Marechal V, Nicand E: Validation of single real-time TaqMan PCR assay for the detection and quantitation of four major genotypes of hepatitis E virus in clinical specimens. J Med Virol 2006; 78:1076–1082.
44 Inoue J, Takahashi M, Yazaki Y, Tsuda F, Okamoto H: Development and validation of an improved RT-PCR assay with nested universal primers for detection of hepatitis E virus strains with significant sequence divergence. J Virol Methods 2006;137: 325–333.
45 Zhang F, Li X, Li Z, Harrison TJ, Chong H, Qiao S, Huang W, Zhang H, Zhuang H, Wang Y: Detection of HEV antigen as a novel marker for the diagnosis of hepatitis E. J Med Virol 2006;78:1441–1448.
46 Tian DY, Chen Y, Xia NS: Significance of serum IgA in patients with acute hepatitis E virus infection. World J Gastroenterol 2006;12:3919–3923.
47 Fukuda S, Sunaga J, Saito N, Fujimura K, Itoh Y, Sasaki M, Tsuda F, Takahashi M, Nishizawa T, Okamoto H: Prevalence of antibodies to hepatitis E virus among Japanese blood donors: identification of three blood donors infected with a genotype 3 hepatitis E virus. J Med Virol 2004;73:554–561.
48 Arankalle VA, Chobe LP: Hepatitis E virus: can it be transmitted parenterally? J Viral Hepat 1999;6: 161–164.
49 Zaaijer HL, Mauser-Bunschoten EP, ten Veen JH, Kapprell HP, Kok M, van den Berg HM, Lelie PN: Hepatitis E virus antibodies among patients with hemophilia, blood donors, and hepatitis patients. J Med Virol 1995;46:244–246
50 Ritter A, Witteler H, Simpson B, Chiewsilp P, Hinde B, Vidler J, Lemair L, Castella D: A multicentre study of HEV seropositivity in random blood donors. J Hepatol 1993;18(suppl 1):25.
51 Bekanntmachung der Richtlinien zur Gewinnung von Blut und Blutbestandteilen und zur Anwendung von Blutprodukten (Hämotherapie) gemäß §§ 12 und 18 des Transfusionsgesetzes (TFG) (Novelle 2005) vom 19. September 2005. Bundesanzeiger 2005, Nr. 209a, 05.11.2005.
52 Bekanntmachung der Richtlinien zur Gewinnung von Blut und Blutbestandteilen und zur Anwendung von Blutprodukten (Hämotherapie) gemäß §§ 12 und 18 des Transfusionsgesetzes (TFG) (Änderungen und Ergänzungen 2007) vom 17. April 2007. Bundesanzeiger 2007, Nr. 92, 19.05.2007, S. 5075.
53 Burger R, Gerlich W, Gürtler L, Heiden M, Hitzler W, Jansen B, Lefèvre H, Löwer J, Ludwig WD, Montag-Lessing T, Neumann R, Paessens A, Pauli G, Seitz R, Schlenkrich U, Werner E, Willkommen H: Hepatitis A virus. Infus Ther Transfus Med 2001; 28:354–360.
54 Mitsui T, Tsukamoto Y, Yamazaki C, Masuko K, Tsuda F, Takahashi M, Nishizawa T, Okamoto H: Prevalence of hepatitis E virus infection among hemodialysis patients in Japan: evidence for infection with a genotype 3 HEV by blood transfusion. J Med Virol 2004;74:563–572.
55 Barzilai A, Schulman S, Karetnyi YV, Favorov MO, Levin E, Mendelson E, Weiss P, Fields HA, Varon D, Martinowitz U: Hepatitis E virus infection in hemophiliacs. J Med Virol 1995;46:153–156.
56 Buti M, Jardi R, Cotrina M, Rodriguez-Frias F, Troonen H, Viladomiu L, Esteban JI, Esteban R, Guardia J: Hepatitis E virus infection in acute hepatitis in Spain. J Virol Methods 1995;55:49–54.
57 Tamura A, Shimizu YK, Tanaka T, Kuroda K, Arakawa Y, Takahashi K, Mishiro M, Shimizu K, Moriyama M: Persistent infection of hepatitis E virus transmitted by blood transfusion in a patient with T-cell lymphoma. Hepatol Res 2007;37: 113–120.
58 Pillot J, Turkoglu S, Dubreuil P, Cosson A, Lemaigre G, Meng J, Lazizi Y: Cross-reactive immunity against different strains of the hepatitis E virus transferable by simian and human sera. C R Acad Sci III 1995;318:1059–1064.
59 Worm HC, Wirnsberger G: Hepatitis E vaccines: progress and prospects. Drugs 2004;64:1517–1531.
60 Maloney BJ, Takeda N, Suzaki Y, Ami Y, Li TC, Miyamura T, Arntzen CJ, Mason HS: Challenges in creating a vaccine to prevent hepatitis E. Vaccine 2005;23:1870–1874.
61 Deshmukh TM, Lole KS, Tripathy AS, Arankalle VA: Immunogenicity of candidate hepatitis E virus DNA vaccine expressing complete and truncated ORF2 in mice. Vaccine 2007;25:4350–4360.
62 Dong C, Dai X, Meng JH: The first experimental study on a candidate combined vaccine against hepatitis A and hepatitis E. Vaccine 2007;25: 1662–1668.
63 Shrestha MP, Scott RM, Joshi DM, Mammen MP, Thapa GB, Thapa N, Myint KS, Fourneau M, Kuschner RA, Shrestha SK, David MP, Seriwatana J, Vaughn DW, Safary A, Endy TP, Innis BL: Safety and efficacy of a recombinant hepatitis E vaccine. N Engl J Med 2007;356:895–903.

Transfusion Medicine and Hemotherapy

Transfus Med Hemother 2009;36:48–60
DOI: 10.1159/000197327

Malaria

Arbeitskreis Blut, Untergruppe «Bewertung Blutassoziierter Krankheitserreger»

1 Current Knowledge about the Pathogen

Malaria occurs world-wide in more than 100 countries in the tropical and subtropical regions and is the most significant parasitic disease in humans. Each year, it causes disease in approximately 500 million people and kills between 1 and 3 million people, above all children under 5 years. Four different types of protozoae are responsible for the disease. They belong to the genus *Plasmodium* (class haematozoea, order haemosporida). These include:

- *Plasmodium falciparum* – the agent of tropical malaria
- *Plasmodium vivax* und *Plasmodium ovale* – the agent of tertian malaria.
- *Plasmodium malariae* – the agent of quartan malaria.

P. falciparum consists of genetically different types and, based on the analyses of core and mitochondria nucleic acid sequences, is the agent most closely related to *Plasmodium gallinaceum*. It probably originates from Africa [1]. As can be derived from the mutations found, the age of *P. falciparum* is estimated to be 10,000–100,000 years which corresponds to the evolution of the hominids since in Central and North Europe no markers can be found for selection pressure by malaria [2]. Humans are the only hosts for these four human pathogenic *Plasmodium* species. In rare cases, infections are caused by malaria parasites of other primates (e.g. *Plasmodium knowlesi, Plasmodium cynomolgie* and *Plasmodium simium*).

1.1 Characteristics of Malaria

Plasmodium is a parasite that grows intracellularly. The life cycle of plasmodium develops in two phases: an asexual phase in the human host and a sexual phase in the carrier, the *Anopheles* mosquito. The sporozoites transmitted during a blood meal rapidly penetrate from the blood stream into the liver parenchymal cells in which they replicate asexually. Depending on the plasmodium species, this so-called schizogony phase lasts between 5–7 days in *P. falciparum* and between 6–18 days in the other species. Schizogony, formerly referred to as merogony, is the asexual replication of the protozoae. A schizont contains several cell nuclei; the daughter nuclei are surrounded by cytoplasm and organise themselves into single individuals, the merozoites. One single sporozoite can produce between 10,000 and more than 30,000 merozoites. For *P. vivax* and *P. ovale*, part of the schizonts remain in a kind of inactive phase (hypnozoites); they can remain in the liver cell for months or years, and may then lead to the relapses characteristic of tertian malaria.

After schizogony is completed, the swollen liver cell ruptures and releases the mobile merozoites into the blood stream. These adhere to the red blood cells via specific surface receptors (receptor in the case of *P. vivax* e.g. Duffy blood group antigen, Fy^a or Fy^b, or in case of *P. falciparum* glycophorin A). Then, they enter the red blood cells and turn into trophozoites. At the end of the 48- to 72-hour erythrocytic phase, the schizonts will have formed in the red blood cells. During this phase, so-called seal-ring shapes (vacuoles with parietal nuclei) may form (cf. fig. 1). From decayed red blood cells, new merozoites may be released which can infect further red blood cells. A part of the merozoites differentiates within erythrocytes into sexual stages, forming macro- and microgametocytes. In the intra-erythrocytic vacuoles, haemozoin is formed as an insoluble metabolite of haemoglobin, called malaria pigment.

After ingestion of male and female gametocytes during a blood meal, a motile flagellated zygote is formed in the midgut of the *Anopheles* mosquito. This zygote moves into the salivary gland. An oocyst is formed releasing sporozoites which can infect a new human host via the saliva of the mosquito.

1.2 Infection and Infectious Disease [3–5]

Malaria infection in humans is caused by a sting of the female *Anopheles* mosquito during which sporozoites are released

KARGER

Fax +49 761 4 52 07 14
Information@Karger.de
www.karger.com

Accessible online at:
www.karger.com/tmh

Previously published in Transfus Med Hemother 2008;35:122–134

from the salivary gland of the mosquito into the organism of the host during a blood meal. The sporozoites then go through the cycle described in 1.1 'Characteristics of Malaria'. The symptoms in humans are caused by the invasion and destruction of the red blood cells by the asexual parasites and the immune response of the host. The red blood cells are affected by strong consumption and degradation of intracellular proteins, especially of haemoglobin, caused by the growing parasites. Changes occur in the membrane of the red blood cell, and their deformability is reduced. Above all, the adhesion protein PfEMP-1 (*P. falciparum* erythrocyte membrane protein-1) plays an important part in the pathogenesis of *P. falciparum*. This protein mediates the adherence to the receptors of the venous and capillary endothelium (cell adherence). Around 60 different var-genes encode for different variants of PfEMP-1, each with individual antigenic and adhesive properties.

It is assumed that one particular PfEMP-1 each is prevalent on the surface of one individual infected red blood cell. Receptor molecules for PfEMP-1 above all include the intercellular adhesion molecule 1 (ICAM-1) in the brain, chondroitin sulphate B in the placenta, and CD36 in other organs. Infected red blood cell can also adhere to other non-affected red blood cells (rosette formation) and other infected red blood cells (agglutination). Cell adhesion and rosette formation will lead to sequestration of the red blood cells which contain mature forms of the parasite in the capillaries of different organs (especially the brain). The impairment of microcirculation, caused by the cell adherence of the red blood cells amongst each other and the cell adherence to the endothelium, the resulting reduction of blood flow in the capillaries, the possible intravasal coagulation activation and the changes in the metabolism will lead to reduced oxygen supply in the brain, kidneys, liver and lungs, which are responsible for the severe course and deadly complications of tropical malaria.

The symptoms of acute malaria are non-specific and begin no sooner than 6 days after a sting by an infected mosquito during the intraerythocytic phase of the development cycle. The symptoms which first occur include malaise, headache, abdominal pain, limb and muscle pain as well as fever. Frequent symptoms are nausea, vomiting, diarrhoea, and orthostatic hypotension. In case of tropical malaria caused by *P. falciparum*, the fever occurs irregularly while symptomatic phases with chills and fever in 48- or 72-hour cycles occur in case of infections with *P. vivax, P. ovale* or *P. malariae* (tertian or quartan malaria). Individuals who are not immune may develop body temperatures of 40 °C and higher. In many cases, thrombopenia is present, and in addition, splenomegaly and hepatomegaly as well as diarrhoea in 30% of the cases.

If tropical malaria is left untreated or is inappropriately treated, complicated malaria can develop in different organs due to sequestration of infected red blood cells. Characteristic phenomena for such complicated courses of tropical malaria include impairments of consciousness up to coma, often in connection with seizures (cerebral malaria), hypoglycaemia, lactic

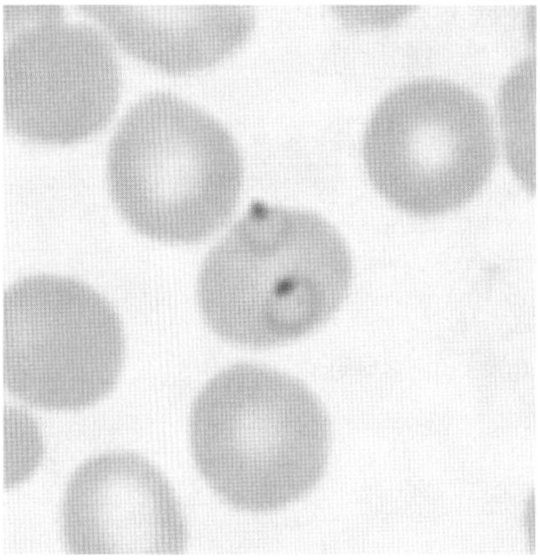

Fig. 1. *Plasmodium falciparum* ring shapes in thin blood smear.

acidosis, impairment of the kidney and liver functions, ARDS (adult respiratory distress syndrome) and haematological changes, especially pronounced haemolytic anaemia. In addition, coagulation disorders (only very seldom as disseminated intravasal coagulation), thrombocytopenia and haemoglobinuria may occur. The pathogenetic mechanisms underlying the symptoms of tropical malaria are only partly known and include disorders of the microcirculation (cerebral malaria, impairment of the kidney function), anaerobic glycolysis (lactic acidosis), haemolysis (anaemia) and disorders of the metabolism such as reduced gluconeogenesis in the liver, hyperinsulinaemia and increased glucose consumption by parasites (hypoglycaemia).

The most severe course of tropical malaria is cerebral malaria. This is the course which is in most cases responsible for the high lethality, despite appropriate treatment, and for neurological deficits, especially in children. During pregnancy, tropical malaria is related to increased maternal and foetal morbidity and lethality. In semi-immune primigravid and secundigravid women, cerebral malaria results in low birth weight and increased infant and child mortality due to reduced oxygen supply. An HIV infection of the mother predisposes for increased parasitaemia and increases the risk of connatal malaria. In non-immune pregnant women, the risk of infection with severe outcome and high parasitaemia and anaemia is high. Severe tropical malaria, as a rule, leads to a miscarriage. Connatal malaria occurs in less than 5% of the newborns of infected mothers in endemic areas.

The clinical course of tropical malaria in children resembles that of adults. Above all in infants more than 6 months of age, who no longer have a certain protection from malaria by maternal antibodies, and in small children, the course is often serious with a high complication rate in contrast to adults, with serious anaemia causing cerebral malaria. According to WHO estimates, more than half the estimated 1–3 million annual deaths in African children is caused by tropical malaria.

Clinical symptoms of tertian malaria caused by *P. vivax* resembles tertian malaria caused by *P. vivax*. Both parasites infect only young red blood cells (reticulocytes) so that parasitaemia

Table 1. Time from end of travel up to the occurrence of symptoms in cases of malaria reported in accordance with the IfSG (Infection Protection Act) who did not stay in the country of travel for longer than 8 weeks

Form of malaria	Number of cases from 2001–2006	Number of cases with information on end of travel and beginning of symptoms	Months after end of travel	Portion of cases with symptoms, %
Tropical	3,334	1,446	2	98.8
			6	99.8
			12	99.9
			13	100
Tertian	796	261	2	55.6
			6	85.4
			12	97.7
			60	100
Quartan	103	33	2	81.8
			6	100

in the blood is detectable in only 1–2% of the red blood cells. Symptoms that may occur include anaemia due to haemolysis, thrombocytopenia and in rare cases rupture of the spleen. Microcirculatory disorders due to sequestration of the red blood cells may also occur very seldom.

Because of the occurrence of dormant parasite forms in the liver (hypnozoites), relapses can occur after remitting tertian malaria after up to 4 years. In extreme cases, even longer relapse periods were observed.

Quartan malaria which is caused by *P. malariae* as a rule has a benign course with only mild symptoms. The parasites infect predominantly old red blood cells; the result is low parasitaemia (1–2%) in the blood, as in tertian malaria. Glomerulonephritis due to chronic formation of immune complexes with deposits in the kidney may occur. Unlike tertian malaria, quartan malaria displays no hypnozoites in the liver and therefore no latent hepatic courses. Late quartan malaria attacks (recrudescences) may result from persisting forms of *P. malariae* in blood vessel endothelia [5]. Quartan malaria can persist for up to 40 years.

Chronic complications of malaria include the tropical splenomegaly syndrome, the nephrotic syndrome in case of quartan malaria and possibly an increased occurrence of Epstein-Barr virus (EBV) associated Burkitt lymphoma during childhood.

1.3 Epidemiology

According to the WHO, there were possible transmissions of malaria in a total of 107 countries in 2004 [6]. Although this figure has declined since the 1950s (140 countries with endemic malaria), roughly 3.2 billion people currently live at a permanent risk of malaria. It is estimated that every year between 350 and 600 million clinical cases of malaria occur world-wide, out of which 60% occur in Africa south of the Sahara alone. Out of the more than 1 million deaths in Africa caused by malaria, roughly half are children under 5 years.

Almost all of these deaths are due to tropical malaria. *P. falciparum* mainly occurs in Africa and in certain regions of South-East Asia, the Caribbean and South America. The second most frequent malaria species, *P. vivax*, is found in wider parts of Asia, America, and North Africa. Altogether, more than 40 different *Anopheles* mosquito species are able to transmit malaria. The most important malaria vector, *Anopheles gambiae*, occurs exclusively in Africa.

The extent of endemic occurrence of malaria is calculated from the degree of parasitaemia or the rate in children between 2 and 9 years with an enlargement of the spleen. If the rate is below 10%, we talk about hypoendemic, between 11 and 50% about mesoendemic, between 51 and 75% of hyperendemic and with a portion of spleen enlargements of over 75% of holoendemic regions. In certain holo- and hyperendemic regions of tropical Africa or New Guinea with a very high transmission rate of *P. falciparum*, the inhabitants are repeatedly infected with plasmodia throughout their lifetime. In these regions, there is a high morbidity and mortality during childhood. Whereas health impairments are serious in children, malaria infections in adults frequently show few symptoms because of the adult's partial immunity. Such a situation with frequent re-infections throughout the entire year is described as 'stable malaria' and occurs in holo- and hyperendemic regions. In hypoendemic regions, the transmission rate is low, and infections only occasionally occur seasonally or in certain districts. Depending on external circumstances (e.g. rainy season), the incidence of malaria can be markedly increased, and epidemics can occur. In general, the epidemiology of malaria is influenced by the number of infectious stings, the mosquito density, the number of infected mosquitoes, the number of chronically infected individuals, the degree of anthropophilia of the vector, the interval between the blood meals, the lifetime of the mosquitoes and the sporozoite infection dose. The ambient temperature also plays an important role, since development of human pathogenic plasmodia persists below 16 °C. Thus, an endemic spread of *P. vivax* as occurred about 100 years ago in Central Europe is no longer possible since the human host is missing thanks to a successful treatment of malaria.

In Germany, altogether 628 cases of malaria were reported in 2005 pursuant to the § 7 IfSG (Infektionsschutzgesetz; German Infection Protection Act). This corresponds to an incidence of 0.8 cases of infection per 100,000 inhabitants. In the years before 2005, the reported figures were 707 cases (2004), 820 cases (2003), 859 cases (2002), 1,045 cases (2001), 836 cases (2000), 931 cases (1999), and 1,008 cases (1998) [7]. The largest portion of malaria infections in 2005 was imported from African countries (88%). 7% of the reported cases originated from Asia, 3% from America, and 2% from Australia/Oceania. Among those countries from which malaria was imported, Ghana, Nigeria, Cameroon and Kenya were at the top of the list. In 78% of the malaria cases reported in 2005, *P. falciparum* was identified as the agent of tropical malaria while *P. vivax* ranked second with 12%, and *P. ovale* and *P. malariae* were registered with only 4 and 3%. Among the total of 6 deaths by tropical malaria in 2005, three cases had infection with *P. falciparum*, one case had a mixed infection, and in 2 cases no pathogen species was identified. One of the individuals originated from Cameroon, and 5 were German. Evidence showed that 2 of the individuals who died had not performed chemoprophylaxis. The countries of origin indicated were Cameroon, Gambia, Senegal and Ghana.

Out of the cases of malaria reported to the Robert Koch Institute for 2001 to 2006 (as of 12 July 2007), altogether 4,639 cases fulfilled the reference definition. For part of the cases reported, both the time of travel and the onset of symptoms of the disease were available. Although no exact incubation period can be derived from these data, the time of the onset of clinical symptoms after returning from an endemic area is important for blood safety concerns, i.e. the determination of deferral periods. This especially applies to infection with *P. vivax* and *P. ovale* as well as *P. malariae*, since these may have longer incubation periods. An analysis of the data on individuals who did not stay in an endemic area for malaria for more than 8 weeks (individuals who do not have their temporary centre of activity there), shows that in 14.6% of the returnees reported on tertian malaria in accordance with the IfSG symptoms occurred only after more than 6 months (table 1). Similar information was also obtained from Switzerland [8].

The rare cases of malaria infections acquired in non-endemic areas are either transfusion associated malaria cases (cf. 3 'Recipients') or so-called airport malaria and/or nosocomial transmissions. Airport malaria is transmitted during the flight or a stop-over and/or by mosquitoes e.g. transported in the luggage [9]. Nosocomial malaria transmissions can be caused e.g. by needle injuries, contaminated fluids and contaminated medical devices [10–13].

Besides, autochthonous malaria transmissions (i.e. transmissions which developed on site) can occur in regions in which malaria does not usually exist or has been eradicated if the respective vector is present (*Anopheles* spp.). Thus, 7 locally restricted transmissions of *P. vivax* were reported in Palm State County, FL, USA, in 2003 [14].

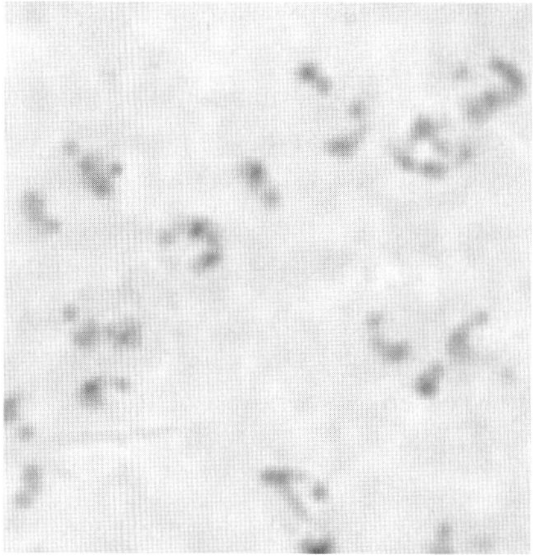

Fig. 2. *Plasmodium falciparum* ring shapes in thick drop.

Anopheles spp. native to Germany, too, can transmit plasmodia; depending on ambient temperature, infectious chains are therefore well possible in Germany and have occurred before. *P. vivax* and tertian malaria were wide-spread in Southern Germany up to the middle of the 19th century. At the Upper Rhine, malaria did not recede before the straightening of the Rhine which reduced the breeding grounds for *Anopheles*. Sporogeny of *P. vivax* in *Anopheles* occurs up to a summer isotherm of 16 °C. The main areas of distribution are within the 25 °C summer isotherm which runs through the middle of Germany [15]. In the past few decades, no case of endemic malaria has been reported in Germany. The last autochthonic cases of malaria were observed up to around 1950 in Berlin and its surroundings [16].

Malaria caused by *P. falciparum* has recently been reported in 2 German children, who had no history of international travels but stayed at a hospital at the same time as a child from Angola infected with tropical malaria. Since breeding grounds of *Anopheles plumbeus* (a potential plasmodium carrier) were found in the vicinity of the hospital and, in addition, temperatures were between 21 and 27 °C on average during the day time, transmission by *A. plumbeus* was assumed as the possible cause [17].

1.4 Detection Methods and Their Significance

1.4.1 Thick Drop and Blood Smear

The gold standard for malaria diagnostics is still the microscopic examination of the so-called thick drop or thin blood smears stained in accordance with May-Grünwald or Wright-Giemsa, respectively [18], or by means of fluorescence colouring (figs 1, 2). In the thick drop method, plasmodia are enriched to the 6- to 10-fold concentration compared with the blood smear. The degree of parasitaemia/µl can be determined by means of the parasite and leucocyte count via a correlation with the total leucocyte count. A negative test result does not reliably exclude a malaria infection since at the beginning of clinical manifestation the parasite density might be low in the peripheral blood. In case of continued clinical suspicion and negative results, the test must be repeated several times, e.g. at 12-hour intervals. The experience of the investigator plays an important part in malaria diagnostics. The detection limit is 5–10 parasites/μl. In the case of less experienced investigators, it is increased to the power of 10.

1.4.2 NAT Method

Various investigators have compared in particular the sensitivity of NAT tests with conventional microscopy after staining in accordance with Giemsa or Wright-Giemsa. All studies showed a higher sensitivity after DNA extraction by means of NAT. Around 5–10 μl blood are used for blood smear or thick drop; for DNA extraction, the quantity is 200 μl.

For the conventional nested PCR, different primers are used to include all plasmodia species. These primers bind in the 18s RNA [19, 20]. Sensitivity of microscopy is approximately 93% if 100% are set in the PCR. Other methods included real-time PCR [21] and real-time PCR with probes as molecular beacon [22]. An arithmetic sensitivity of 0.004 parasites/μl blood was obtained for *P. falciparum*, and for genus-specific PCR this figure was 0.16/μl [22]. Compared with microscopy, a sensitivity of 97.4% was obtained with genus-specific sensitivity [23]. According to another report, no cross-reaction with *Toxoplasma gondii* and *Leishmania infantum* was found at a sensitivity of 0.7 parasites/μl for *P. falciparum*, 4 parasites/μl for *P. vivax*, and 1.5 parasites/μl for *P. ovale* [24].

1.4.3 Plasmodium Antigen Detection

The first few tests for the determination of plasmodium components showed low sensitivity and specificity [25–27], even though parasitic LDH was used as antigen. Rapid tests were developed to support travellers in malaria diagnostics in the event of fever or exposure. Direct detection tests for plasmodium have been improved in the meantime so that a sensitivity of 85% and a specificity of 96% can be reached for *P. falciparum* infections [28]. Low parasite density could be a reason for low sensitivity. The antibody cross-reacts with *P. vivax*, but at a low sensitivity. When antibodies were used against histidine-rich protein II of *P. falciparum*, a sensitivity of 97% and a specificity of 96% were obtained in travel returnees [29].

Depending on the exposure, a sensitivity of 88% and a specificity of 99% can be reached for *P. falciparum*. For *P. vivax*, the respective figures are 76% and 100%[30]. Monoclonal antibody based ELISA has shown a sensitivity of 90% for *P. falciparum* in Thailand and Nepal [31].

The quality of the plasmodium indicated in each study quoted depends on the comparative tests used in these studies, i.e. PCR or microscopy, and on the investigator's expertise in interpreting the test result.

1.4.4 Diagnostics Using Anti-Plasmodium Antibodies

Most of the studies published in this field deal with the determination of antibodies which are formed after a vaccination or which can be used for the appropriate antigens for a putative vaccine. The cytoadherence-linked asexual gene 9 (clag 9) [32], merozoite surface proteins 6 and 7 (MSP6, MSP7) [33] and the variant surface antigens (VSA) are immunogenic and can still be detected 10 years after infection [34].

Exposure to malaria parasites which was measured via IgM and IgG responses using a test containing 5 different proeryrthocyte antigens was published by some working groups from France in 2006. The test antigens were circumsporozoite protein, sporozoite threonine- and asparagine-rich protein, sporozoite and liver stage antigen, liver stage antigen 1 and SR11.1. The immune response was measured in 106 individuals 3 months after exposure and seemed plausible [35]. If leucin-rich protein is used, cross-reactions occur between *Schistosoma mansoni* and *P. falciparum* [36].

Since the infection with *P. falciparum* in the blood causes serious clinical symptoms, the testing of returnees from tropical regions after a delay of several months in the case of an asymptomatic state of health is immaterial from an epidemiological point of view. Testing for anti-plasmodium antibodies has more informational value as regards the exposure and possible circulation if no clinical abnormality has shown.

2 Blood and Plasma Donors

2.1 Prevalence and Incidence in Donor Populations

Little is known about the prevalence and incidence of malaria in blood donors in Germany. In an up-to-date study by Okocha et al. [37], a prevalence of antibodies of 30.2% was determined in donors in Nigeria. In Venezuela, 890 blood donors were studied by Nunez et al. [38] by means of ELISA. The total antibody prevalence found was 1.7%.

2.2 Definition of Exclusion Criteria

Conforming to the guidelines of the Bundesärztekammer (German Medical Association) on haemotherapy, individuals in Germany are excluded from donating blood for a period of 4 years following medically documented recovery from malaria [39]. In addition, persons who were born or raised in a malaria endemic area or temporarily had their centre of life in such an area are deferred from donating blood for a total of 4 years after their last stay in the endemic area. Before donating blood, infectiveness has to be excluded by means of a validated immunological or nucleic acid test. Persons visiting a malaria endemic area for a short period are not allowed to donate blood for a period of at least 6 months following their stay. The decision of a possible deferral is independent from the occurrence of febrile episodes. For persons exclusively donating plasma for fractionation, exclusion from the donation due to a malaria risk need not be considered.

In the UK, potential donors who had a malaria infection or fever of unclear origin within 6 months after returning from an endemic area, or after having stayed in a malaria endemic area during the past 12 months or for an uninterrupted period of more than 6 months, are excluded from the donation. A negative test result for anti-plasmodium antibodies is required for re-admittance to the donor panel 3 years after the end of treatment or after 6 months free of symptoms after returning from the endemic area [40].

In France, antibody tests (indirect immunofluorescence antibody test; IFAT) are also performed within a period of between 4 months and up to 3 years after returning from an endemic area. The test algorithm depends on the duration of the stay in the malaria endemic area.

2.3 Donor Testing and Significance

Because of existing exclusion rules, no donor screening for plasmodium is carried out in Germany.

2.4 Donor Interviews

In countries with endemic occurrence of malaria in which a high portion of the donors is infected, the kind of donor exclusion which is common practice in non-endemic countries cannot be performed because a lack of donated blood supply would result. Besides, a great number of recipients have partial immunity. In some malaria endemic countries, recipients received administrations of chloroquine or, in the event of chloroquine resistance, sulfadoxin-pyrimethmin in order to prevent transfusion associated malaria. However, this type of preventative measure is not reliable in the very regions of Central and West Africa as well as South-East Asia due to increased resistance against these two substances.

When potential donors in Germany are interviewed, they are asked whether they originated or grew up in a malaria endemic region or whether they stayed in such a region in the past 6 months. A possible malaria prophylaxis is not taken into account here. In addition, the donor is obliged to indicate whether he/she has an acute malaria infection or ever had a malaria infection.

2.5 Donor Information and Counselling

Information or advice for a donor concerning malaria is not provided. If the donor is suspected to be infected with malaria, further clarification by a physician experienced in tropical medicine is required.

3 Recipients

3.1 Prevalence and Incidence of Blood-Associated Infections and Infectious Diseases in Recipient Populations

The first transmission of malaria by blood transfusion was described in 1911 in a patient with pernicious anaemia [41]. Although the donor indicated that he had never suffered from malaria, the recipient developed a febrile reaction 11 days following the donation, and *P. vivax* could be detected both in the donor and in the recipient. More than roughly 350 malaria infections following blood transfusions were reported for the years between 1910 and 1950 [42]. An analysis of the cases that became known between 1911 and 1979 [43] showed an increase in the incidence of malaria from 6 to 145 cases per year, parallel to the increasing number of transfusions. At first, *P. vivax* was the most frequently observed species in case of transfusion associated malaria while *P. malariae* prevailed in the 1950s. In the 1970s, *P. vivax* was again the prevalent species in cases of transfusion associated malaria followed by *P. malariae* and *P. falciparum*. Since the 1980s, however, *P. falciparum* has been the most frequently registered species of malaria following blood transfusions in countries in which malaria does not occur endemically (e.g. USA, Canada and UK). Thus, the portion of *P. falciparum* in the UK has risen from 37% in 1984 to 55% in 1993 [44].

Altogether 93 cases of transfusion associated malaria have been documented in the USA during the period from 1963 to 1999 [45]. 35% could be ascribed to *P. falciparum*, 27% to *P. vivax*, 27% to *P. malariae*, 5% to *P. ovale* and 3% to mixed infections. 11% of the patients died. Of 91 identified donors altogether, 67 could be associated with the transmission. 59% of the donors whose country of origin was known came from endemic areas. The estimated incidence of transfusion associated malaria in the USA is one case per 1 million donors. Around 1–3 cases per year are reported in the US Center for Disease Control and Prevention (CDC). It is assumed that the frequency of transfusion associated malaria in malaria endemic countries is more than 50 cases per 1 million donors. In Canada, the frequency of transfusion associated malaria is estimated to be 1 case per 4 million transfused red blood cell concentrates [46]. The three cases of tropical malaria published in 2001 were all transmitted by donors originating from malaria endemic areas but had lived in Canada symptom free for several years. Based on these 3 cases, the Canadian donor deferral criteria were amended to exclude persons who had recovered from malaria (2 of the 3 cases) permanently from donation.

Up to 1965, a total of 12 cases of transfusion associated malaria were reported from Germany [47–53]. The cases in question were 2 infections with *P. falciparum* and 7 infections with *P. vivax*, the 3 remaining infections could not be reliable assigned [overview in 42].

In the past few years, 3 reports were published on transfusion associated cases of malaria [54–56]. In 1998, Witt et al. [56] reported on an 18-month-old boy who developed antibiotic refractory fever 14 days after a heart operation. On day 23, postoperative, intraerythrocytic ring shapes and gametocytes of *P. falciparum* were found in the peripheral blood smear. The child recovered rapidly after a 3-day administration of quinine and halofantrine. The retrospective analysis of the deferred samples of 7 donors from which the child had received red blood cell concentrates showed antibodies against *P. falciparum* in one of the donors.

Malaria caused by *P. falciparum* with lethal outcome was recently reported from a 70-year-old patient after preceding operation due to coronary heart disease and aortic aneurysm which was caused by transfusion of red blood cell concentrates. One of the blood donors was a 30-year-old man born in Cameroon who had left the country 10 years before and had ever since lived in Paris (near the International Airport) and later on in Switzerland. His last visit to his home country had been 6 years back at the time of the medical investigations. A possible cause of the infection of the donor was assumed to be airport malaria or persistence with partial immunity [57].

3.2 Immune Status (Resistance, Existing Immunity, Immune Response, Age, Exogenous Factors) [3, 4]

The course of malaria strongly depends on the degree of immunity of the infected individual. Complete sterile immunity is never reached, but merely partial immunity (semi-immunity). Immunity is proportional to the age, the cumulative number of malaria episodes and time spent continuously in a malaria endemic region.

Based on transplacentally transmitted maternal antibodies, newborns have a certain degree of immunity to malaria up to an age of around 4–6 months, whereby foetal haemoglobin inhibits maturing of the schizonts. Older children and young adults in regions with stable malaria and a high transmission rate (holoendemic or hyperendemic regions) possess the highest degree of immunity. Here, asymptomatic parasitaemia can often be found. In semi-immune individuals – polyclonal increase in IgM, IgG and IgA antibodies as well as specific T-lymphocytes can act cytotoxically against parasites or infected cells in the liver. The most important antigen in infections with *P. falciparum* is probably variable protein PfEMP-1. The acquisition of antibodies against a number of variant PfEMP-1 antigens seems to be of special significance for the immunity situation. Specific immunity is directed both against the species and against the respective subpopulation of the parasites.

Non-immune individuals only have the non-specific defence mechanisms, and the course of tropical malaria in such individuals is by far more severe than in semi-immune persons.

Congenital red blood cell anomalies also play an important role in immunity to malaria. In malaria endemic areas, hereditary diseases such as sickle cell anaemia, thalassaemia or glucose-6-phosphate dehydrogenase deficiency of the red blood cells can be found. In individuals with heterozygoty of HbAS (sickle cell gene carriers), there is a certain immunity against tropical malaria. This seems to be due to the inhibited growth of the parasites caused by strongly reduced oxygen content. Higher resistance can also be found in heterozygote α-thalassaemia. Glucose-6-phosphate dehydrogenase deficiency is also associated with reduced susceptibility to malaria in children and pregnant women and is caused by inhibition of growth of the parasites in red blood cells in which the latter enzyme is missing. Ovalocytosis, which occurs in South-East Asia, leads to lower parasitaemia in heterozygote carriers.

Red blood cells where the Duffy blood group antigen Fy^a is missing are partly resistant to *P. vivax*. This is how the very low incidence of malaria caused by *P. vivax* in West Africa can explained, where a high percentage of the population does not possess the Duffy blood group antigen Fy^a [58].

3.3 Severity and Course of the Disease

Untreated tropical malaria always has a fatal outcome in non-immune individuals who do not originate from an endemic area.

In a US study performed on transfusion associated malaria from the years 1963–1998 with a total of 93 cases, a lethality rate of 11% (10 cases) was observed [45]. Six of these patients had an infection with *P. falciparum*, 2 were infected with *P. vivax*, and 2 with *P. malariae*. The two patients with *P. vivax* died of their underlying disease.

Out of 5 patients with post-transfusion malaria in the UK [59], 1 died of cerebral tropical malaria and another *P. falciparum* infected patient died of multiple organ failure. In another study [60], lethality of transfusion associated malaria is indicated as 15%. No figures are available from Germany. The high lethality rate of transfusion associated malaria can be explained by the fact that most of the cases documented are cases of immunologically naïve recipients with a more or less serious underlying disease, or this rare route of infection was diagnosed too late.

The incubation period of transfusion associated malaria depends on the species and the number of transmitted parasites, and is between 10 and 60 days [43]. For *P. falciparum*, it is 10 days on average, for *P. vivax* 16 days, and for *P. malariae* 40 days [42]. Symptoms of transfusion associated malaria are many and varied. They include dizziness, vomiting, muscle pain, slight icterus, abdominal pain and diarrhoea. Usually, no fever periodicity can be found. In patients with serious underlying disease, above all immune suppression, transfusion associated malaria often displays a severe course with early cerebral involvement.

Table 2. Overview of products for malaria prophylaxis and stand-by treatment for malaria (modified in accordance with the recommendations from the *Deutsche Gesellschaft für Tropenmedizin und Internationale Gesundheit* (DTG, German Society for Tropical Medicine and International Health)

Product	Prophylaxis	Stand-by treatment
Chloroquine	300 mg chloroquine base weekly – for persons > 75 kg body weight: 450 mg weekly – 1 week before up to 4 weeks after a stay in a malaria area	600 mg base, 6 h after the beginning of treatment and 300 mg at a time 24 and 48 h after the beginning of treatment
Mefloquine	250 mg weekly, 1–3 weeks before up to 4 weeks after a stay in a malaria area	Initial dose 750 mg, after 6–8 h further 500 mg; if body weight >60 kg after another 6–8 h further 250 mg
Atovaquone-proguanil	250 mg/100 mg daily, 1–2 days before up to 7 day after a stay in a malaria area (adults with a body weight > 40 kg; maximal duration of stay 28 days)	1,000 mg / 400 mg as a single dose on 3 subsequent days if the body weight is > 40 kg
Doxycyclin	100 mg daily 1–2 days before and up to 4 weeks after a stay in a malaria area	not suitable
Artemether-lumefantrine	not suitable	80 mg / 480 mg initial dose after 8 h further 80 mg / 480 mg, then 2× daily 80 mg / 480 mg on days 2 and 3
Proguanil	200 mg daily	not suitable

3.4 Therapy and Prophylaxis

3.4.1 Vaccine Development

Although a variety of attempts have been made to develop effective malaria vaccines, practically no immunisation is commercially available yet [61]. In the past few years, malaria has been recognised as a global social problem, and intensive activities are underway to develop new vaccines, which is to a considerable extent the merit of the generous funding from the European Union and the Bill and Melinda Gates Foundation. The number of clinical trials is on the increase so that new vaccines can be expected in the next few years. The distribution of roles between humoral and cell-bound factors in effective immunity against plasmodia, however, is not understood [58].

The development work focuses on vaccines against *P. falciparum* and/or tropical malaria as the most dangerous form of malaria. Four stages of the life cycle of *P. falciparum* are eligible as targets of immune prophylaxis in humans:

- sporozoites after a blood meal or before infection of the hepatocytes,
- the merozoites after release from the liver or before invasion of the red blood cells,
- the merozoites during invasion of the red blood cells or replication in the red blood cells, and
- the gametocytes released from the red blood cells in the anopheles mosquito after the next blood meal [61].

The overwhelming majority of the development studies focus on potential vaccines which are intended to prevent the invasion in the red blood cells, and thus the massive replication of the parasites. It is expected that this would inhibit the clinical symptoms of malaria, and above all, the complications relating to these symptoms. If the red blood cell stage could be completely blocked, this would automatically break the infection chain which would also be significant from an epidemiological point of view. Strictly speaking, only vaccines against sporozoites preventing the invasion of the liver cell and leading to the killing of parasites should be considered as causal immune prophylaxis. Such variants, however, will probably not be a subject of discussion in the near future, due to the complexity of the parasites and the number of unresolved scientific problems. From the transfusion medicine point of view, we must bear in mind that, even if a donor is protected by a vaccination, it should not automatically be assumed that no transfusion related malaria will occur. What is more relevant here is to calculate this risk taking into account the epidemiological and infectiological background and the type of immune protection.

3.4.2 Prophylaxis and Therapy

Primary prevention of malaria is brought about by mosquito bite prevention. Other preventative measures include the reduction of the parasite reservoir in the population in malaria endemic regions, measures to eradicate vectors (removal of breeding grounds, use of larvicides, and insecticides), as well as measures to reduce contact with the vector.

Attempts have been made to immunise the *Anopheles* mosquito against the parasite in order to break the infection chain. Travellers to malaria endemic areas are still strongly recommended to undergo exposure prophylaxis, e.g. the use of repellents, wearing clothes that provide protection, sleeping under mosquito netting and staying in mosquito proof rooms. In addition, chemoprophylaxis is recommended depending on the destination and the type of travel. Depending on the resistance situation, the Deutsche Gesellschaft für Tropenmedizin und Internationale Gesundheit (DTG; German Society for Tropical Medicine and International Health) recommends chloroquine, mefloquine, atovaquone-proguanil, or, in some cases, doxycyclin for malaria prophylaxis (table 2) [62]. In this context, the distinction is made between continued chemopro-

Table 3. Treatment of malaria, modified in accordance with [63]

	Product	Dosage
Malaria tertiana Malaria quartana	chloroquine	10 mg base/kg body weight initial dose, followed by 5 mg base/kg body weight after 6, 24, and 48 h
	plus primaquine (only in case of tertian malaria)	0.5 mg base/kg body weight 1 × daily over a period of 14 days
Malaria tropica		
Non-complicated malaria	mefloquine	initially 750 mg base, followed by 500 mg base 6 h after the beginning of treatment and 250 mg base 12 h after the beginning of treatment (at >60 kg body weight)
	or atovaquone-proguanil	1,000 mg/day atovaquone, 400 mg/day proguanil 1 × daily over a period of 3 days
	or arthemether-lumefantrine	80 mg / 480 mg arthemether-lumefantrine initial dose, followed by 80 mg / 480 mg arthemether-lumefantrine after 8 h, 2 × 80 mg / 480 mg arthemether-lumefantrine on day 2, 2 × 80 mg / 480 mg arthemether-lumefantrine on day 3
Complicated forms	quinine salt (quinine-dihydrochloride)	3 × 10 mg p.inf./kg body weight/day for 7–10 days
	plus doxycyclin	3 mg/kg body weight/day for 7 days

phylaxis (which as a rule begins one week or day before travelling to the malaria area and continues up to 4 weeks or 1 week after leaving the malaria area, depending on the situation), and the stand-by treatment with the appropriate medicine (mefloquine, atovaquone-proguanil, artemeter-lumefantrine). The use of halofantrin for malaria prophylaxis was stopped in Germany many years ago because of its risk of cardiac adverse effects.

In pregnant women, the use of a combination of chloroquine and proguanil is possible as from the second trimester. For children primarily consistent exposure prophylaxis is recommended. Prophylaxis with atovaquone-proguanil is possible for children with a body weight ≥11 kg while mefloquine can be used in children with a body weight over 5 kg. Doxycyclin must not be used in children under 8 years of age. However, chemoprophylaxis does not guarantee that the patient will be free from malaria, but will reduce the risk significantly.

Because of the world-wide occurrence of e.g. chloroquine and sulfadoxin-pyrimethamine resistent isolates of *P. falciparum*, meloqine, atovaquone-proguanil, or arthemether-lumefanine are now the treatments of choice in non-complicated tropical malaria. Treatment of serious tropical malaria (with CNS involvement, acute kidney failure or other organ complications) should be performed under intensive-ward conditions at all means. Treatment with medicinal products usually consists of parenteral administration of quinine in combination with doxycyclin.

Due to the still relatively favourable resistance situation, chloroquine is still the treatment of choice in tertian malaria. After completion of the chloroquine course of treatment, completion treatment with primaquine which is efficacious against hypnozoites of *P. vivax* and *P. ovale* should follow. Quartan malaria should also be treated with chloroquine. Subsequent treatment with primaquine is not required (table 3). The same principles as for general malaria treatment apply for treatment of transfusion associated malaria, except that in infections caused by *P. vivax* and *P. ovale*, no subsequent treatment with primaquine is required because a liver cycle, i.e. hypnozoites, is not involved in this type of infection (cf. 1.2. 'Infection and Infectious Disease'). In this type of infection, too, it is early start of treatment which is decisive for the outcome. Prophylaxis is currently possible only by strict exclusion criteria for donors, in combination with serological and/or molecular biology screening (NAT) if required. A vaccination which confers protection is so far not available.

3.5 Transmissibility

A risk of transmissibility of malaria by transfusion exists because of the primary presence of parasites in red blood cells, above all in transfusion of whole blood or red blood cells. However, there is also a risk of transmission with platelet concentrates [64], leucocyte concentrates [65], and even fresh frozen plasma; the latter has only been observed with the administration of fresh frozen plasma within one day following collection [66]. Three infections with malaria were described due to non-observance of the basic principles of hygiene [67] or needle perforation injury [10, 68], and three other transfusion associated cases of malaria recently were described in Canada [46]. These give rise to the assumption that even low numbers of infected red blood cells can cause malaria infection.

Due to the long survival times in the human organism (e.g. *P. malariae*), a donor can still have malaria parasites in the blood after years and can cause an infection in the recipient. In general, *P. vivax* and *P. ovale* rarely persist longer than 3 years while *P. falciparum* persists about 1–2 years. The longest intervals between blood donation and malaria exposure of the donor in the past were 13 years in the case of a *P. falciparum* infection [69], 27 years for a *P. vivax* infection [69] and 7 years in a *P. ovale* infection [70]. For *P. malariae*, considerably longer time intervals have been described – in an extreme case – up to 50 years or even more.

3.6 Frequency of Administration, Type and Amount of Blood Products

For plasma derivatives, contamination with plasmodia can be excluded thanks to the manufacturing procedure.
In principle, transmission is possible with only one single product of a non-pathogen-inactivated blood component since all products show residual red blood cell contents.

4 Blood Products

4.1 Infectious Load of the Starting Material and Test Methods

Most donors involved in the cases of transfusion associated malaria are semi-immune individuals with low parasitaemia in the blood. As is known from previous studies, plasmodia can survive in blood reserves for at least 10–12 days, possibly longer [43, 71]. Apparently, the minimum infective dose in humans is 10 parasites (for *P. vivax*) [65]. In the case of assumed (low) parasitaemia in the donor of 1–2 parasites per µl blood, however, as many as 250,000–500,000 parasites would be transmitted if 250 ml red blood cell concentrate was donated. Methods for detecting a potentially infected donation which would have to contain as few as 10 parasites, would have to be able to detect as little as 0.00004 parasites per µl blood [43, 72]. This degree of sensitivity is not even achieved with the NAT method.
The test methods usually applied for malaria such as microscopic examination of 'thick drop' or blood smear in accordance with Giemsa (sensitivity for both methods between 5–500 parasites/µl blood) are not suitable for donor screening because of the usually very low parasitaemia of the donor. Antigen tests based on the detection of HRP/2 or pLDH, too, only detect between 100 and 1,000 parasites/µl blood. Compared with that, NAT methods display higher sensitivity [73, 74]. In a study [75], as little as 0.004 parasites/µl blood could be detected in potentially malaria exposed donors. However, NAT is not able to detect all potentially infectious donors, even at this high sensitivity.

Targeted serological examination of donors returning from malaria endemic areas has been successfully performed in France since 1983. After a deferral period of 4 months, donors are tested using the IFAT. If the result is negative, the donor can be re-admitted. No transfusion associated case of malaria became known in France between 1984 and 2002 [76]. Disadvantages of the IFAT however, include its limitation to antibodies against *P. falciparum* with low cross-reactivity against the other plasmodia species, high workload in the laboratory and its poor reproducibility due to the subjective assessibility of the test method. Enzyme immunoassays have recently been developed, partly also with recombinant antigens [44, 72]. Thus, a combination of donor interviewing and testing with enzyme immunoassays with recombinant antigen is currently recommended in England for reducing the malaria risk after blood transfusion.

4.2 Methods for Removal and Inactivation of the Infectious Agent

For plasma derivatives, transmission of malaria can be excluded thanks to the manufacturing procedure. Therefore, no cases of malaria due transmission of fractionated plasma products have so far been described.

4.3 Feasibility and Validation of Procedures for Removal/ Inactivation of the Infectious Agent

Some papers have recently been published on the inactivation of plasmodia in blood components by means of different methods (gamma irradiation, photochemical and photodynamic inactivation) [77–81], but without being able to establish whether these methods can be considered as sufficiently reliable and without being considered as routine procedures up to now. In contrast to that, the INTERCEPT system for pathogen inactivation in platelet concentrates and plasma for transfusion is currently beginning to become established in the blood bank routine of some countries. This photochemical method in which the photoactive compound amotosalen HCI is added to the blood components which are at the same time irradiated with long-wavelength UV light (UVA) has proven to be effective for *P. falciparum* by showing a pathogen reduction of >6 log levels [82].

5 Assessment

With by far more than 1 billion people affected, malaria, which occurs in the world's tropical and subtropical areas, is one of the most significant parasitary infections in humans. The protozoae, which are transmitted by the sting of the female *Anopheles* mosquito, (*P. falciparum*, *P. vivax*, *P. ovale* and *P.*

malariae) cause different forms of malaria in humans. Tropical malaria which is caused by *P. falciparum* is the infection mainly responsible for the 1–3 million deaths occurring per year world-wide, and out of which more than half are African children.

In Germany, the number of malaria infections reported in the past few years varies between around 600 and 1,000 cases per year. These are caused by travelling, very rarely by importing infected *Anopheles* (airport malaria) and in very isolated cases by autochthonous infections.

Depending on the resistance situation, medicinal products such as chloroquine, mefloquine, atovaquone-proquanil, or doxycyclin are used for chemical malaria prophylaxis. Donors are deferred independently from such a malaria prophylaxis. No vaccination is currently commercially available which confers protection against malaria.

During the period up to 1965, altogether 12 cases of transfusion associated malaria became known in Germany. Three reports on malaria following blood transfusions in Germany are available in the literature from a more recent time. Since the Paul Ehrlich Institute became responsible for blood products (1994), one single case of transfusion associated malaria was reported from 1997.

To prevent transfusion associated malaria, persons are excluded from donating blood after medically documented cure from malaria for a period of 4 years. In addition, persons who were born or grew up or temporarily had there centre of life in a malaria endemic area are excluded from donating blood for 4 years following their stay in the endemic area. Returnees from a malaria endemic area are currently deferred from donating blood for a minimum of 6 months following their last stay in a malaria endemic area. If only plasma for fractionation is donated, no exclusion from the donation based on a malaria risk is required.

Altogether, this risk of transfusion associated malaria is considered as low in Germany. A high standard of safety is guaranteed thanks to the thorough investigation of the history of the patient and donor selection as well as the exclusion criteria used for returnees from tropical areas. New epidemiological data for Germany show that with the current referral period of 6 months after travels to endemic areas not all plasmodia infections are detected, especially infections with *P. vivax* or *P. ovale*, since in 15% of the cases reported, symptoms occur only after that period. An extension of the deferral period to 12 months would include nearly 99% of the malaria infections. An argument against an extension of the deferral period and the loss of donors relating to this would be the fact that there has so far been no case of transmission since the introduction of the 6-month regulation. If the epidemiological situation changes, however, the deferral period will have to be reviewed and adjusted.

Even though testing of blood donors for malaria antibodies or the presence of plasmodium antigens or for plasmodium genome by means of the NAT method is laid down in the 'Richtlinien zur Gewinnung von Blut und Blutbestandteilen und zur Anwendung von Blutprodukten (Hämotherapie)' (Guidelines for the collection of blood and components from blood, as well as for the use of blood products (haemotherapy)) [39] for donors before re-admittance as donor after the 4-year deferral, no tests are commercially available guaranteeing the detection of antibodies against all four human pathogenic *Plasmodium* spp., which would, however, be imperative for diagnostics with informational value. The inactivation of plasmodia in blood components, which is feasible in principle, should not be required as a general method for Germany because of the low malaria prevalence. Concerning this issue as well as concerning the development of a suitable vaccine, extensive research is certainly required in order to optimise the safety for recipients of blood and blood products regarding malaria.

This paper was completed on March 19, 2007 and approved by the German Advisory Committee Blood (Arbeitskreis Blut) on October 1, 2007. It was compiled by the members of the subgroup 'Assessment of Pathogens Transmissible by Blood' of the German Advisory Committee Blood (Arbeitskreis Blut):

Dr. Johannes Blümel
Prof. Dr. Reinhard Burger
Prof. Dr. Christian Drosten
Dr. Albrecht Gröner
Prof. Dr. Lutz Gürtler
Dr. Margarethe Heiden
Prof. Dr. Dr. Bernd Jansen
Dr. Horst Klamm
Prof. Dr. Wolf-Dieter Ludwig
Dr. Thomas Montag-Lessing
Dr. Ruth Offergeld
Prof. Dr. Georg Pauli
Prof. Dr. Rainer Seitz
Dr. Uwe Schlenkrich
Dr. Volkmar Schottstedt
Dr. Hannelore Willkommen
Prof. Dr. Karl-Heinz Wirsing von König
with special support by Prof. Dr. Jürgen Knobloch (University of Tübingen)

References

1 Conway DJ: Molecular epidemiology of malaria. Clin Microbiol Rev 2007;20:188–204.
2 Hartl DL: The origin of malaria: mixed messages from genetic diversity. Nature Rev Microbiol 2004;2:15–22.
3 Fairhurst R, Wellems T: Plasmodium species (malaria); in Mandell G, Bennett G, Dolin R (eds): Principles and Practice of Infectious Diseases. Philadelphia, Elsevier Churchill Livingstone, 2005, pp 3121–3144.
4 Zoller T, Suttorp N: Malaria und Babesiose: Parasitäre Erkrankungen der Erythrozyten; in Dietel M, Suttorp N, Zeitz M (Hrsg): Harrisons Innere Medizin. Berlin, ABW Wissenschaftsverlag, 2005, pp 1309–1323.

5 Kretschmer H, Bienzle U, Klauß V, Kremsner P, Leichsenring M: Malaria; in Knobloch J (Hrsg): Tropen- und Reisemedizin. Jena, Gustav Fischer, 1996, pp 134–163.

6 WHO: World Malaria Report 2005. *http://rbm.who.int./wmr2005*.

7 Robert Koch-Institut: Reiseassoziierte infektionsbedingte Erkrankungen im Jahr 2004. Epidemiol Bull 2005;35:317–324.

8 Lehky Hagen MR, Haley TJ, Christoph Hatz FR: Factors influencing the pattern of imported malaria. J Travel Med 2005;12:72–79.

9 Mouchet J: Airport malaria: a rare disease still poorly understood. Eurosurveillance 2000;5:75–80.

10 Alweis RL, DiRosario K, Conidi G, Kain KC, Olans R, Tully JL: Serial nosocomial transmission of *Plasmodium falciparum* malaria from patient to nurse to patient. Infect Control Hosp Epidemiol; 2004;25:55–59.

11 Moro ML, Romi R, Severini C, Casadio GP, Sarta G, Tampieri G, Scardovi A, Pozzetti C; Malaria Outbreak Group: Patient-to-patient transmission of nosocomial malaria in Italy. Infect Control Hosp Epidemiol 2002;23:338–341.

12 Piro S, Sammud M, Badi S, Al Ssabi L: Hospital-acquired malaria transmitted by contaminated gloves. J Hosp Infect 2001;47:156–158.

13 Chen KT, Chen CJ, Chang PY, Morse DL: A nosocomial outbreak of malaria associated with contaminated catheters and contrast medium of a computed tomographic scanner. Infect Control Hosp Epidemiol 1999;20:22–25.

14 Centers for Disease Control and Prevention (CDC): Local transmission of *Plasmodium vivax* malaria. – Palm Beach County, Florida, 2003. MMWR Morb Mortal Wkly Rep 2003;52(38): 908–911.

15 Lucius R, Frank B: Parasitologie. Heidelberg, Spektrum Akademischer Verlag , 1997.

16 Fischer L: Einheimische Malaria und Anophelismus in der Nachkriegszeit. Dtsch Med Wochenschr 1948;73:515–518.

17] Krüger A, Rech A, Xin-Zhuan S, Tannich E: Two cases of autochthonous *Plasmodium falciparum* malaria in Germany with evidence for local transmission by indigenous *Anopheles plumbeus*. Trop Med Intern Health 2001;6:983–985.

18 Warhurst DC, Williams JE: ACP Broadsheet no 148, July 1996. Laboratory diagnosis of malaria. J Clin Pathol 1996;49:533–538.

19 Snounou GS, Viriyakosol S, Zhu XP, Jara W, Pinheiro L, do Rosario VE, Thaithong S, Brown KN: High sensitivity of detection of human malaria parasites by the use of nested polymerase chain reaction. Mol Biochem Parasitol 1993;61:315–320.

20 Johnston SP, Pieniazek NJ, Xayavong MV, Slemenda SB, Wilkins PP, da Silva AJ: PCR as a confirmatory technique for laboratory diagnosis of malaria. J Clin Microbiol 2006;44:1087–1089.

21Malhotra I, Dent A, Mungai P, Muchiri E, King CL: Real-time quantitative PCR for determining the burden of *Plasmodium falciparum* parasites during pregnancy and infancy. J Clin Microbiol 2005;43(8): 3630–3635.

22 Elsayed S, Plewes K, Church D, Chow B, Zhang K: Use of molecular beacon probes for real-time PCR detection of *Plasmodium falciparum* and other *Plasmodium* species in peripheral blood specimens. J Clin Microbiol 2006;44:622–624.

23 Mangold KA, Manson RU, Koay ESC, Stephens L, Regner MA, Thomson RB, Peterson LR, Kaul KL: Real-time PCR for detection and identification of *Plasmodium* spp. J Clin Microbiol 2005;43: 2435–2440.

24 Perandin F, Manca N, Calderaro A, Piccolo G, Galati L, Ricci L, Medici MC, Arcangeletti MC, Snounou G, Dettori G, Chezzi C: Development of a real-time PCR assay for detection of Plas*modium falciparum, Plasmodium vivax,* and *Plasmodium ovale* for routine clinical diagnosis. J Clin Microbiol 2004;42:1214–1219.

25 Grobusch MP, Alpermann U, Schwenke S, Jelinek T, Warhurst DC: False-positive rapid tests for malaria in patients with rheumatoid factor. Lancet 1999;353:297.

26 Hänscheid T, Valadas E: Poor accuracy of rapid diagnostic tests and misdiagnosis of imported malaria: are PCR-based reference laboratories the answer? J Clin Microbiol 2002;40:736–737.

27 Mankhambo L, Kanjala M, Rudman S, Lema VM, Rogerson SJ: Evaluation of the OptiMal rapid antigen test and species-specific PCR to detect placental *Plasmodium falciparum* infection at delivery. J Clin Microbiol 2002;40:155–158.

28 Playford EG, Walker J: Evaluation of the ICT malaria P.f/P.v and the OptiMal rapid diagnostic tests for malaria in febrile returned travellers. J Clin Microbiol 2002;40:4166–4171.

29 Richardson DC, Ciach M, Zhong KJY, Crandall I, Kain KC: Evaluation of the Makromed dipstick assay versus PCR for diagnosis of *Plasmodium falciparum* malaria in returned travelers. J Clin Microbiol 2002;40:4528–4530.

30 Jelinek T, Grobusch MP, Harms G: Evaluation of a dipstick test for the rapid diagnosis of imported malaria among patients presenting within the network TropNetEurop. Scand J Infect Dis 2001;33: 752–754.

31 Joshi HH: Monoclonal antibody based ELISA: an effective diagnostic tool for the diagnosis of falciparum malaria. J Nep Med Assoc 2005;44:79–83.

32 Trenholme KR, Boutlis CS, Kuns R, Lagog M, Bockarie MJ, Gatton M, Kemp DJ, Good MF, Anstey NM, Gardiner DL: Antibody reactivity to linear epitopes of *Plasmodium falciparum* cytoadherence linked asexual gene 9 in asymptomatic children and adults from Papua New Guinea. Am J Trop Med Hyg 2005;72:708–713.

33 Wang L, Crouch L, Richie TL, Nhan DH, Coppel RL: Naturally acquired antibody responses to the components of the *Plasmodium falciparum* merozoite surface protein 1 complex. Parasite Immunol 2003;25:403–412.

34 Nielsen MA, Vestergaard LS, Lusingu J, Kurtzhals JAL, Giha HA, Grevstad B, Goka BQ, Lemnge MM, Jensen JB, Akanmori BD, Theander TG, Staalsoe, Hviid L: Geographical and temporal conservation of antibody recognition of *Plasmodium falciparum* variant surface antigens. Infect Immun 2004;72(6):3531–3535.

35 Orlandi-Pradines E, Penhoat K, Durand C, Pons C,Bay C, Pradines B, Fusai T, Josse R, Dubrous P, Meynard JP, Durand JP, Migliani R, Boutin JP, Druilhe P, Rogier C: Antibody responses to several malaria pre-erythrocytic antigens as a marker of malaria exposure among travelers. Am J Trop Med Hyg 2006;74:979–985.

36 Pierrot C, Wilson S, Lallet H, Lafitte S, Jones FM, Daher W, Capron M, Dunne DW, Khalife J: Identification of a novel antigen of *Schistosoma mansoni* shared with *Plasmodium falciparum* and evaluation of different cross-reactive antibody subclasses induced by human schistosmiasis and malaria. Infect Immun 2006;74:3347–3354.

37 Okocha EC, Ibeh CC, Ele PU, Ibeh NC: The prevalence of malaria parasitaemia in blood donors in a Nigerian teaching hospital. J Vector Borne Dis 2005;42:21–24.

38 Nunez L, Linares J, Perez AH: Seroprevalence of antibodies against *Plasmodium falciparum* in volunteer donors from various cities in Venezuela. Sangre (Barc) 1992;37(2):141–143.

39 Bundesärztekammer: Richtlinien zur Gewinnung von Blut und Blutbestandteilen und zur Anwendung von Blutprodukten (Hämotherapie) gemäß §§ 12 und 18 des Transfusionsgesetzes (Novelle 2005). Bundesanzeiger 2005;57 (Nr.209a).

40 Joint UKBTS / NIBSC Professional Advisory Committee: Whole Blood & Components Donor Selection Guidelines. *http://www.transfusionguidelines.org.uk/index.asp?Publication=WB*.

41 Woolsey G: Transfusion for pernicious anemia: two cases. Ann Surg 1911;53:132–134.

42 Bruce-Chwatt LJ: Blood transfusion and tropical disease. Trop Dis Bull 1972;69:825–862.

43 Bruce-Chwatt LJ: Transfusion malaria revisited. Trop Dis Bull 1982;79:827–840.

44 Chiodini PL, Hartley S, Hewitt PE, Barbara JA, Lalloo K, Bligh J, Voller A: Evaluation of a malaria antibody ELISA and its value in reducing potential wastage of red cell donations from blood donors exposed to malaria, with a note on a case of transfusion-transmitted malaria. Vox Sang 1997;73:143–148.

45 Mungai M, Tegtmeier G, Chamberland M, Parise M: Transfusion-transmitted malaria in the United States from 1963 through 1999. N Engl J Med 2001; 344:1973–1978.

46 Slinger R, Giulivi A, Bodie-Collins M, Hindieh F, John RS, Sher G, Goldman M, Ricketts M, Kain KC: Transfusion-transmitted malaria in Canada. CMAJ 2001;164:377–379.

47 Oehlecker F: Übertragung latenter Malaria bei direkter Bluttransfusion. Dtsch Med Wochenschr 1920;46:1025–1026.

48 Schnitzler H: Übertragung von latenter Malaria tertiana durch Bluttransfusion. Zentralbl Chir 1929; 56:1438.

49 Majanz A: Beiträge zur Frage der Bluttransfusion. Dtsch Z Chir 1930;224:171–185.

50 Stohlmann H: Malariaübertragung auf Blutspende. Münch Med Wochenschr 1943;90:84–85.

51 Menk W: Bluttransfusion und Malaria. Münch Med Wochenschr 1944;91:349–350.

52 Lampen H: Induzierte Malaria nach Bluttransfusion. Med Klin 1947;42:371–372.

53 Mohr W: Malariaübertragung durch Bluttransfusionsgerät. Med Klin 1950;45:94.

54 Nolte K, Stibbe W, Kuhlencord A, Bommer W, Gallasch E: Transfusionsbedingte Malaria tropica. Beitr Infusionsther Klin Ernähr 1987;18:42–46.

55 Schunkert H, Handt S, de Wit M, Gladziwa U, Glöckner W, Sieberth H: Transfusionsmalaria bei Promyelozytenleukämie. Dtsch Med Wochenschr 1988;113:1841–1843.

56 Witt O, Iglauer A RJ, Bommer W, Eber S: Transfusionsmalaria als Ursache von unklarem postoperativen Fieber. Monatsschr Kinderheilkd 1998; 146:1054–1056.

57 Frey-Wettstein M, Maier A, Markwalder K, Munch U: A case of transfusion transmitted malaria in Switzerland. Swiss Med Wkly 2001;131:320.

58 Knobloch, Jürgen (Hrsg): Malaria – Grundlagen und klinische Praxis. Bremen, Unimed, 2003.

59 Kitchen AD, Barbara JA, Hewitt PE: Documented cases of post-transfusion malaria occurring in England: a review in relation to current and proposed donor-selection guidelines. Vox Sang 2005;89:77–80.

60 Guerrero IC, Weniger BG, Schultz MG: Transfusion malaria in the United States, 1972–1981. Ann Intern Med 1983;99:221–226.

61 Graves P, Gelband H: Vaccines for preventing malaria. Cochrane Database Syst Rev 2006 (2 und 4): CD000129.
62 Deutsche Gesellschaft für Tropenmedizin und Internationale Gesundheit (DTG): Empfehlungen zur Malariavorbeugung, 2006. *www.dtg.org/Malaria. html.*
63 Leitlinie der AWMF (Association of the Medical Societies in Germany): Diagnostik und Therapie der Malaria. Leitlinienregister Nr. 042/001.
64 Garfield MD, Ershler WB, Maki DG: Malaria transmission by platelet concentrate transfusion. JAMA 1978;240:2285–2286.
65 Dover AS, Guinee VF: Malaria transmission by leukocyte component therapy. JAMA 1971;217: 1701–1702.
66 Lazner E, Newhouser E: Studies on the transmission of malaria by blood transfusions. Am J Med Sci 1943;204:141–146.
67 Al-Saigul AM, Fontaine RE, Haddad Q: Nosocomial malaria from contamination of a multidose heparin container with blood. Infect Control Hosp Epidemiol 2000;21:329–330.
68 Winterberg DH, Wever PC, Rheenen-Veerberg CV, Kempers O, Durand R, Bos AP, Teeuw AH, Spanjaard L, Dunkert J: A boy with nosocoial malaria tropica contracted in a Dutch hospital. Ped Infect Dis J 2005;24:89–91.
69 Besson P, Robert JF, Reviron J, Richard-Lenoble D, Gentilini M: 2 cases of transfusional malaria. Attempted prevention combining an indirect immunofluorescence test with clinical selection criteria. Rev Fr Transfus Immunohematol 1976;19: 369–373.
70 Nahlen BL, Lobel HO, Cannon SE, Campbell CC: Reassessment of blood donor selection criteria for United States travelers to malarious areas. Transfusion 1991;31:798–804.
71 Bruce-Chwatt LJ: Transfusion malaria. Bull World Health Organ 1974;50:337–346.
72 Seed CR, Kitchen A, Davis TM: The current status and potential role of laboratory testing to prevent transfusion-transmitted malaria. Transfus Med Rev 2005;19:229–240.
73 Moody A: Rapid diagnostic tests for malaria parasites. Clin Microbiol Rev 2002;15:66–78.
74 Vu TT, Tran VB, Phan NT, Le TT, Luong VH, O'Brien E, Morris GE: Screening donor blood for malaria by polymerase chain reaction. Trans R Soc Trop Med Hyg 1995;89:44–47.
75 Benito A, Rubio JM: Usefulness of seminested polymerase chain reaction for screening blood donors at risk for malaria in Spain. Emerg Infect Dis 2001;7:1068.
76 Silvie O, Rubinstein E, Franetich JF, Prenant M, Belnoue E, Rénia L, Hannoun L, Eling W, Levy S, Boucheix C, Mazier D: Hepatocyte CD81 is required for *Plasmodium falciparum* and *Plasmodium yoelii* sporozoite infectivity. Nat Med 2003;9: 93–96.
77 Smith TG, Kain KC: Inactivation of *Plasmodium falciparum* by photodynamic excitation of hemecycle intermediates derived from delta-aminolevulinic acid. J Infect Dis 2004;190:184–191.
78 Zavizion B, Serebryanik D, Chapman J, Alford B, Purmal A: Inactivation of Gram-negative and Gram-positive bacteria in red cell concentrates using INACTINE PEN110 chemistry. Vox Sang 2004;87:143–149.
79 Ferreira-da-Cruz MF, Teva A, Espindola-Mendes EC, dos Santos LG, Daniel-Ribeiro CT: Inactivation of *Plasmodium falciparum* parasites using gamma-irradiation. Mem Inst Oswaldo Cruz 1997; 92:137–138.
80 Grellier P, Santus R, Mouray E, Agmon V, Maziere JC, Rigomier D, Dagan A, Gatt S, Schrével J: Photosensitized inactivation of *Plasmodium falciparum* and *Babesia divergens*-infected erythrocytes in whole blood by lipophilic pheophorbide derivatives. Vox Sang 1997;72:211–220.
81 Lustigman S, Ben Hur E: Photosensitized inactivation of *Plasmodium falciparum* in human red cells by phthalocyanines. Transfusion 1996;36:543–546.
82 Singh Y, Sawyer LS, Pinkoski LS, Dupuis KW, Hsu JC, Lin L, Corash L: Photochemical treatment of plasma with amotosalen and long-wavelength ultraviolet light inactivates pathogens while retaining coagulation function. Transfusion 2006;46:1168–1177.

Transfusion Medicine and Hemotherapy

Transfus Med Hemother 2009;36:62–78
DOI: 10.1159/000197341

Arbobacteria – Pathogens Transmittable by Arthropods

Arbeitskreis Blut, Untergruppe «Bewertung Blutassoziierter Krankheitserreger»

Anaplasma phagocytophilum, marginatum; Bartonella henselae; Borrelia burgdorferi, afzelii, garinii; Coxiella burnetii; Ehrlichia chaffeensis; Francisella tularensis; Rickettsia prowazekii, akari, rickettsii and*Yersinia pestis* are also known as arbobacteria. Diseases caused by these bacteria are basically zoonoses, i.e. diseases transmittable from animals to humans, and have been known as such for about 100 years (table 1). A part of the individual pathogens have not been described until the past few decades. Based on molecular biology analyses, *R. prowazekii, Ehrlichia* and *Anaplasma* are categorised as Rickettsiales, while *Bartonella* is categorised as alpha-2-proteobacteria, *Coxiella, Rickettsia grylli* and *F. tularensis* as gamma proteobacteria, and *Y. pestis* as enterobacteria [1].

Most arbobacteria grow predominantly intracellularly. However, *Borrelia* bacteria grow intracellularly and extracellularly, and *Yersinia* mainly extracellularly. The above described arbobacteria, when transmitted by ticks, show seasonal occurrence and a partly changed antigen repertoire in vector and mammal. *R. prowazekii* is transmitted by lice world-wide throughout the year.

The major clinical symptoms such infections have in common include fever, exanthema, headache, and lymph node swelling, partly a pronounced erythema at the site of the sting, and encephalitic disorders. Neutropenia and thrombocytopenia can occur later.

Treatment: Doxycycline is the treatment of choice against most of these bacteria, followed by chloramphenicol and cephalosporins. Quinolones are ineffective against *R. prowazekii.* The treatment of choice against *Y. pestis* and *F. tularensis* is streptomycin or gentamycin, and in addition doxycycline or ciprofloxacine.

C. burnetii has been dealt with separately [2]. Therefore, this pathogen is not included in the present review, neither are rare tropical and/or pure tropical diseases. The oriental flea (*Xenopsylla cheopsis*) is considered as the most effective transmitter for *Y. pestis*. More than 30 other flea species are known which can transmit *Y. pestis* as intermediary hosts, including Pulex irritans (human flea), which can play a role in human-to-human transmission. The human louse can also be a vector for transmission of *Y. pestis* [3].

The following section provides for each pathogen information on the general state of knowledge, characteristics of the pathogen, infectious disease, epidemiology, methods of detection and occurrence of the pathogen in the donor population. This is followed by information concerning all pathogens on epidemiology, defence situation, treatment and prevention in recipient populations as well as a summary evaluation.

1 *Anaplasma* and *Ehrlichia*

1.1 Current Knowledge about the Pathogen

Today, after separation into *Ehrlichia* and *Anaplasma*, the pathogens are subdivided as follows:

- *Anaplasma*: A phagocytophilum, platys, marginale.
- *Ehrlichia*: *E. chaffeensis*, with horse as the major host and infection in humans, as well as *Ehrlichia ewingii* and *Ehrlichia canis*, with dog as the major host, which seldom infect humans.

Up to 1987, an *Ehrlichia* infection was considered as a pure animal disease. Ehrlichiosis in dog was first described in Algeria in 1935 with the characteristic inclusions in monocytes in the Giemsa staining. The first infections in humans were reported as Sennetsu Neorickettsiosis in Japan and Malaysia. The first description of the disease after a tick bite in the USA (Arkansas) was done in 1986 [4].

In 1994, *A. phagocytophilum* was described as a distinct pathogen and the disease human granulocytotropic anaplasmosis (HGA) ascribed to it [5].

KARGER

Fax +49 761 4 52 07 14
Information@Karger.de
www.karger.com

Accessible online at:
www.karger.com/tmh

Previously published in Transfus Med Hemother 2008;35:374–390

Table 1. Vectors for arbobacteria

Bacteria	Transmission by				
	Tick(s)	Mosquito	Louse	Flea	Smear infection
Anaplasma *Ehrlichia*	*A. phagocytophila* *E. chaffeensis* *E. ewingii*				
Bartonella		*B. bacilliformis* (*Lutzomyia* as vector)	*B. quintana*	*B. henselae* (cat flea)	*B. henselae* *B. quintana* *B. bacilliformis*
Borrelia	*B. burgdorferi* *B. afzelii* *B. garinii*		*B. recurrentis*		
Coxiella	*C. burnetii*				*C. burnetii*
Francisella	*F. tularensis*	*F. tularensis*			*F. tularensis*
Rickettsia	*R. rickettsii* *R. conorii* *R. slovaca* *R. helvetica*		*R. prowazekii*	*R. typhi*	
Yersinia			*Y. pestis* (experimentally)	*Y. pestis* (*Xenopsylla cheopsis*, rat flea)	*Y. pestis* from open buboes and in case of plague pneumonia (also droplet infection)

1.1.1 Characteristics of the Pathogen

1.1.1.1 Structure

Both pathogens are small Gram-negative bacteria, growing intracellularly and forming inclusion bodies. The pathogen infects both human and animal cells and forms so-called morula cells if excessive growth occurs. Two forms of bacteria can be distinguished – a larger reticular form and a small form with a thick and dense cell wall. The cell wall does not contain any lipopolysaccharides. The surface porin proteins which are present in the wall can be coded by many genes and form the basis for antigen variability of the pathogens. Adhesins for mammalian cells are present, which contain hypervariable regions and carry a very variable portion of sugars so that re-infection with the same, immunologically different bacterium is possible.

1.1.1.2 Replication

Anaplasma and *Ehrlichia* replicate in cells of nymphs and adult ticks, mammals such as deer, cattle and horse as well as humans. In the blood, *Anaplasma* is mainly found in neutrophil granulocytes, macrophages and monocytes, seldom in lymphocytes, whereas *Ehrlichia* predominantly grows in monocytes and macrophages.
Ehrlichia shows a direct cytopathogenic effect in cell culture, to which part of the clinical manifestation can be ascribed. *Anaplasma* cannot be degraded within the neutrophil granulocytes. Apoptosis of these cells is delayed so that bacteria can be replicated over a period of several weeks.

1.1.2 Infection and Infectious Disease

After penetrating the skin, the pathogens grow and spread in white blood cells, and the infection manifests itself in organs such as the liver, spleen, lymph nodes, as well as kidney, lung and brain. Granuloma formation is typical of the disease.
Immune response is inhibited due to intracellular growth, the induced reduction of the number of CD4+, CD8+ and CD5+ cells, and the reduced function of the T lymphocytes. After approximately 30 days, the immune response against the pathogen can be determined via the formation of specific antibodies.
The mean incubation period is 1–4 weeks. The major symptoms of the infection are fever, headache, myalgia and malaise. If the lungs are involved, infiltrates can be detected in the X-ray examination. The average duration of the disease is 9 days, with a range of 1–60 days. Clinical outcome varies from mild symptoms to death. The outcome tends to be more severe at an advanced age of the patients.

1.1.3 Epidemiology

Ehrlichia is transmitted by tick. Transmission reaches its peak from May to August. *Ehrlichia* can be transmitted by the tick species of *Amblyomma americanum*, *Dermatocentor*, and *Ixodes*. *Ehrlichia* infections have mainly been found in North America and South-East Asia. *Anaplasma* is geographically distributed world-wide in regions infested with ticks. Approximately 2% of the ticks in Germany carry *A. phagocytophilum* [6]. Depending on the region, *Ixodes ricinus* ticks carry between 1 and 16% *Ehrlichia* and *Anaplasma*, the highest rates being present in ticks that live in dunes [7].

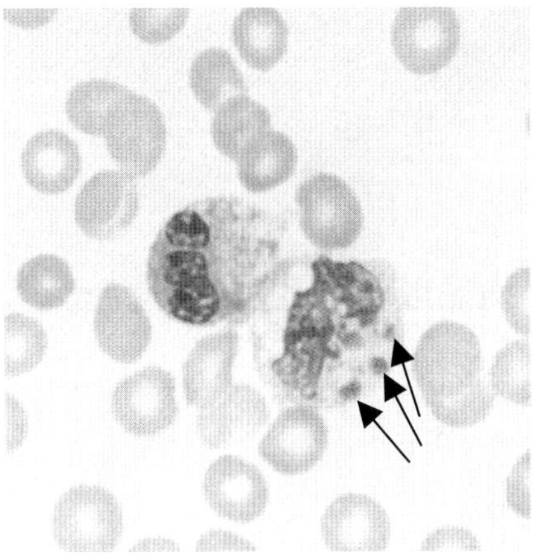

Fig. 1. *Ehrlichia*: Typical dots in mononuclear cells of peripheral blood caused by intracytoplasmic growth of *Ehrlichia* as indicated by the arrows. Shown is a detail of the figure which had been published previously in Clin Microbiol Rev 2003;16:39 [92].

1.1.4 Detection Methods

1.1.4.1 Microscopy and Blood Smear
After Giemsa staining, morulae in *Ehrlichia* can be detected as multiple, round to oval inclusion bodies, measuring 1–3 µm, in the cytoplasm of monocytoid cells of blood and bone marrow (fig. 1). The method is very insensitive, with a sensitivity of approximately 30% [8].

1.1.4.2 NAT
Polymerase chain reaction (PCR) is well suitable for clinical diagnostics. The starting material used most frequently is 16s rRNA, and the primers HE1 and HE3 are used for amplification [9]. Since only few nucleotide exchanges within 1,500 bp of 16s rRNA occur between *Ehrlichia* and *Anaplasma*, distinction between these two pathogens is barely possible using this type of PCR. Specific primers have been developed for the distinction between these species [10].

1.1.4.3 Antibody Detection
Immunofluorescence test slides are commercially available. Immunoblots have been developed to increase specificity [11]. ELISA and immunoblot have been described for *Anaplasma*. Their diagnostic validity remains open. Serological cross-reactivity between *A. marginale* and *A. phagocytophilum* in cattle is 63% [12].

1.2 Blood and Plasma Donors

1.2.1 Prevalence and Incidence in Donor Populations
Up to now, no transfusion-associated transmission of *Anaplasma* or *Ehrlichia* has been reported in Germany. Blood donors are not tested for the presence of *Anaplasma* or *Ehrlichia* bacteria, or antibodies against the latter.
In the USA, *Ehrlichia* has been transmitted via liver and pancreas transplantations [13]. In blood donors with tick bites in endemic areas in the USA, the prevalence of antibodies against *A. phagocytophilum* was 0.9% [14]. An infected tick was also found in the English Garden of Munich [15, 16].

1.2.2 Definition of Exclusion Criteria
The general exclusion criteria apply which point to an infection, such as rise in body temperature, fatigue, exhaustion, muscle pain and anaemia. If applicable, the question should be asked whether a tick bite occurred within the last 4 weeks.

1.2.3 Donor Testing

1.2.3.1 Antibody Determination
Testing for antibodies is not performed. Tests are available (c.f. '1.1.4 Detection Methods').

1.2.3.2 Detection of *Anaplasma* and *Ehrlichia*
Since cultivation requires a very high workload and is expensive but does not show enough sensitivity, PCR is the method of choice, whenever required, (cf. '1.1.4 Detection Methods').

2 *Bartonella*

2.1 Current Knowledge about the Pathogen

The bacterium is named after A.L. Barton who described the intraerythrocytary occurrence of *Bartonella quintana* in 1909. *Bartonella* is the causative agent for the bacillary angiomatosis and the so-called cat-scratch disease. Human pathogen species include *Bartonella bacilliformis, B. henselae* and *B. quintana*. A closer genetic relationship exists with *Brucella* and *Agrobacterium*.
B. bacilliformis only occurs in the Andes of South America at altitudes of between 1,000 and 3,000 m and is transmitted by ticks and midges (species: *Lutzomyia*). Clinical manifestation is known as Oroya fever or Verucca peruana.
B. quintana is transmitted by lice (*Pediculus humanus*) and is found in persons with a low standard of hygiene. The geographical distribution of *B. quintana* is world-wide.
B. henselae also occurs world-wide. Cats seem to be an animal reservoir. In the case of a bacillary angiomatosis, cats very frequently also suffer from bacteraemia. Transmission of *B. henselae* to humans is associated with contact to cats.

2.1.1 Characteristics of the Pathogen

2.1.1.1 Structure
Bartonella is a small 0.6–1.0 µm long Gram-negative rod which can also appear curved. The surface is covered with pili, but no flagellae are present. The bacterium uses the pili e.g. to adhere to endothelial cells.

2.1.1.2 Replication
Bartonella replicates inside and outside human and animal cells, and in the vector. Outside the body, *Bartonella* shows demanding growth. Within the cell, *Bartonella* destroys the cytoskeleton. Infection of endothelial cells is common in all mammals.

2.1.2 Infection and Infectious Disease
The incubation period of *B. quintana* and *B. henselae* is 3–38 days. Acute signs of illness include chills and fever. The fever persists approximately 1–3 weeks. Febrile episodes may take up to 6 weeks. Other manifestations of the disease may include headache, pain in the retrobulbar region, swollen lymph nodes, nystagmus, myalgia, arthralgia and hepatosplenomegaly. Chronic infection with relapsing fever-like episodes may frequently occur in immunocompromised patients. *Bartonella* frequently causes endocarditis. The affected patients are usually afebrile.
Epitheloid angiomatosis manifests itself locally on the skin or in the lymph node. Lesions can be few millimetres or centimetres in diameter and can be similar to Kaposi sarcoma. A typical sign of *Bartonella* is the manifestation of swollen regional lymph nodes. Encephalopathy is very rare as well as death caused by *B. henselae*. Chronic outcome of the disease over several months has only been described in immunosuppressed patients (e.g. by HIV).
Approach to Treatment: Tetracycline, rifampicine and macrolides, preferably azithromycin, are the treatments of choice. In addition, cephalosporins and quinolones may be effective.

2.1.3 Epidemiology
As described above, *B. bacilliformis* only occurs in the South American Andes. The wild animal reservoir for *B. bacilliformis* has not been identified. *B. henselae* and *B. quintana* occur world-wide. Cats are major animal hosts for *B. henselae*. The disease can be prevented by avoiding contact with vectors or cats. Relapses after antibiotic treatment may occur so that a re-occurrence of *Bartonella* infection should not automatically be considered as a new infection.
In Italy, the prevalence of *B. henselae* antibodies in exposed patients has been indicated as 6% [17]. In Swedish elite rangers who stood out due to their occurrence of unexpected cardiac death, the prevalence was 30% for *Bartonella elizabethae*, 3% for *B. henselae* and 1% for *B. quintana* [18].

2.1.4 Detection Methods

2.1.4.1 Antibodies
IgG and IgM Western Blot assays have been developed, with a specificity of 70–95% [19]. The most frequent detection test is performed using immunofluorescence with intracellularly (on Vero-cells) growing *Bartonella* as substrate. Sensitivity is approximately 90%. ELISA is commercially available. High cross-reactivity exists between antibodies against *B. henselae* and those against *B. quintana*.

2.1.4.2 Culturing in Medium
If the transport period to the laboratory is short, *Bartonella* grow in sophisticated culture media such as fresh blood agar and chocolate agar, manifesting themselves as small yellowish, smooth pleomorphic colonies. Blood culture is positive in the case of bacteraemia. *Bartonella* has been isolated from tissues such as liver, spleen, lymph nodes and skin.
Microscopically, Gram-negative rods can be seen but also round shapes.

2.1.4.3 NAT
A PCR method has been described by Handley and Regnery [20] to distinguish between pathogenic *Bartonella* species.

2.2 Blood and Plasma Donors

2.2.1 Prevalence and Incidence in Donor Populations
Bacteriaemia can develop in chronically infected asymptomatic individuals over a long period. A report is available describing the transmission of *Bartonella* by blood transfusion in cats [21]. No studies are available on the prevalence in blood donors in Germany. Transmissions have not been reported.

2.2.2 Definition of Exclusion Criteria
Typical non-specific symptoms of an infection are general exclusion criteria. Skin efflorescence pointing to angiomatosis should be another criterion for temporary donor exclusion.

3 *Borrelia*

3.1 Current Knowledge about the Pathogen

Borrelia is an intracellularly and extracellularly growing Spirochaeta-like bacterium, which occurs world-wide and is essentially transmitted by ticks in North America, Europe and Asia (*Ixodus* and *Dermatocentor* species). The association of tick bite, infection with *B. burgdorferi* and acute Lyme disease was found in 1976 [22]. In 1941, Bannwarth [23] described inflammatory polyneuritis caused by *Borrelia*. Herxheimer and Hartmann [24] described acrodermatitis chronica atrophicans in 1902, and Afzelius [25] described erythema chronicum migrans in 1909.
B. burgdorferi sensu lato is subdivided into 3 pathogenic groups: *B. burgdorferi* sensu strictu, the only strain in Northern America, and in addition, the *B. afzelii* and *B. garinii* groups in Europe. Up until recently, *Borrelia valaisiana* was classified as non-pathogenic.

3.1.1 Characteristics of the Pathogen

3.1.1.1 Structure

Borrelia carries a cytoplasmatic membrane, surrounded with periplasma containing the flagella insertion, and an outer membrane the components of which are not firmly connected with the periplasma. *Borrelia* has a diameter of 0.3–0.5 μm and a length of 8–30 μm. It carries 7–11 flagellae. The linear chromosome is approximately 950 kb in size. Nine circular and 12 linear plasmids contribute to the genome. *Borrelia* contains many lipoproteins such as Osp A to F (outer surface protein) [26]. Various proteins are expressed in different ways during an infection, e.g. VIsE (variable major protein-like sequences expressed) [27] and Salp15 [28].

3.1.1.2 Replication

Borrelia grows both intracellularly and extracellularly on mammalian cell cultures under microaerophilic and anaerobic conditions. *Borrelia* can also be cultured as biopsy material in Barbour-Stoenner-Kelly-II culture medium. Up to now, it has not been possible to achieve replication in solid culture media. The period of generation is 7–20 h at 30–33 °C [29]. Each human cell can be infected, including synovial cells.

3.1.2 Infection and Infectious Disease

Clinical pathogenicity partly derives from the expression of different proteins. Thus, Osp C is barely present in the tick but is highly expressed in the mammal. The same applies to the VIsE. Since these antigens constantly change, the immune response is compromised time and again. Infection occurs by tick bite. 3–32 days later, *Borrelia* replicates in local tissue, usually the skin. *Borrelia* spreads in the body within a few days or weeks, which can lead to bacteriaemia and also infection of the central nervous system. Further preferred replication sites include the myocardium, liver, muscle, retina and spleen.

Osp C, DbpA and DbpB (decorin binding protein), fibronectin binding protein (BBK32 – 47 kDa protein) and VIsE are responsible for the induction of inflammation mediators, depending on the strain.

The disease is subdivided into three stages:

Stage 1 Local Infection: In >50% of the infected individuals, erythema chronicum migrans develops, even though a tick bite is not remembered, since nymphs fall off after feeding on blood. The centre of the erythema may cause a burning or itching sensation and does not necessarily show the characteristic reddening.

Stage 2 Disseminated Infection: After a few days or weeks after the tick bite, multiple lesions develop on the skin as a sign of the haematogenous seed, together with fever, fatigue, exhaustion, and regional lymph node swelling. Meningeal irritation is possible and also hepatitis, splenomegaly, cardiomyopathy, osteomyelitis and panophthalmitis.

Stage 3 Persistent Infection: Months or years after the tick bite, intermittent swelling of the joints, arthritis, axonal neuropathy, encephalomyelitis, with ataxia and cognitive disorders occur, or years after infection, acrodermatitis atrophicans with red painful sclerosing or atrophic induration of the skin. *Borrelia* can be detected in the tissue affected even after long persistence.

Borrelia can be transmitted to the foetus during pregnancy [30].

3.1.3 Epidemiology

In the northern hemisphere, *Borrelia* is wide-spread in North Africa, Europe, including Scandinavia and Russia, China and Japan, and in many other countries. Depending on the endemic area and lifestyle, 1–2% of the population can be infected. Prevalence is higher among forest workers. In the Bavarian Forest e.g. it is 30% [31], and in Italy 7% compared with the general population in the Toscana of 3% [32]. The population in the province around Madrid in Spain also showed an antibody prevalence of 3% [33].

In Southwest and Central Asia, further *Borrelia* strains, e.g. *Borrelia recurrentis*, are transmitted and cause recurrent fever, usually by ticks such as *Ornithodorus* and the lice, *P. humanus*. In Germany, *Borrelia* occurs in all regions in which ticks live. Up to 30% of the ticks can be infected with the 3 species *B. burgdorferi* sensu stricto, *B. garinii* and *B. afzelii*. On average, 11% of the ticks are infected in central and southern Germany. Older ticks have a higher infection rate. The predominant of the three species is *B. garinii* with 60%, followed by *B. burgdorferi* with 32%, and *B. afzelii* with 18% [6]. *B. valaisiana* can occur in 6% of the ticks. Double and few triple infections also occur [6]. In the Netherlands, the infection rate of ticks is between 0.8 and 11.5% [7].

People in all age groups can be infected. Depending on the geographical region, seasonal tick activity in Germany lasts from May to October or from March to November.

3.1.4 Detection Methods

3.1.4.1 Antibodies

The screening test generally used is ELISA, which contains bacterial lysate, recombinant proteins, or a combination of the latter, depending on the manufacturer. IgG and IgM can be detected; IgM can persist over a period of months up to several years. False-positive reactions are not unusual. Therefore, ELISA reactivity is confirmed via immunoblot. Several interpretation criteria have been determined for the immunoblot [34].

3.1.4.2 Indirect Immunofluorescence Assay

The indirect immunofluorescence assay serves as specificity control. Antibodies from patients are absorbed with *Treponema phagedenis*, and then incubated on slides with *Borrelia* cultivated in medium. Antibody titres must be quantitatively evaluated. Experience is required for correct interpretation.

3.1.4.3 Immunoblot
Currently used immunoblot strips are supplemented with recombinant VIsE [27]. The main indication for the use of immunoblots is the clarification of false-positive ELISA results and the serological clarification of neurologic borreliosis.

3.1.4.4 Culturing in Medium
Culturing may be successful in Barbour-Stoenner-Kelly-II medium [29]. This is very time-consuming and requires a high workload on the part of the staff. It is therefore not routinely used.

3.1.4.5 Microscopy
Microscopic analysis shows *Borrelia* as weakly stainable, Gram-negative motile rods. In the blood smear, *B. recurrentis* can normally only be seen during the acute infectious phase.

3.1.4.6 NAT
PCR or derived methods are the methods of choice for the detection of *Borrelia*. PCR can be carried out in all tissues, partly after enriching the 16s DNA.
Sensitivity is between 80 and 95% [35], depending on the primer selection from the Osp A. There is a range of sensitivity between 50–75% dependent on the species, i.e. when *B. burgdorferi* primers are used for the amplification of *B. garinii* or *B. afzelii* Osp A-gene [36].

3.1.4.7 Animal Experiments
Borrelia grows in mice, particularly in the gerbil, and also in rats and hamsters.

3.2 Blood and Plasma Donors

3.2.1 Prevalence and Incidence in Donor Populations
Seroprevalence of blood donors in Germany and Switzerland does not differ from that of the local population. It was 2.7% in Hamburg and Würzburg and 33% in Solothurn [37–39]. Nine blood recipients had no antibodies against *Borrelia* [38] after seroconversion of the donor during follow-up, pointing to low transmission effectiveness. No transmission of *Borrelia* by transfusion has so far been reported in Germany.
In case of bacteriaemia, *Borrelia* can certainly survive at 4 °C during the storage period of the red blood cells, as shown in studies performed by Johnson et al. [40] and by Nadelman et al. [41]. A study in an endemic region such as Connecticut on the risk of *Borrelia* transmission by blood transfusion showed that practically no transmission takes place [42].

3.2.2 Definition of Exclusion Criteria
After *Borrelia* infection by tick bite followed either by local or the usual general signs of inflammation, Lyme disease with its clinical manifestations of fever, fatigue, and exhaustion will be detected by the usual exclusion criteria.
If required, the donor can be asked whether a tick bite occurred within the past 6 weeks, however, this is not a reliable exclusion criterion since, as mentioned above, nymphs fall off after the bite, leaving it unnoticed.

3.2.3 Donor Testing and Significance
To date, blood donors have not been tested routinely for the presence of *Borrelia* antibodies. The current epidemiological situation still does not justify general donor screening for *Borrelia* [38].

3.2.3.1 Antibody Determination
Borrelia antibody determination using ELISA is very sensitive if an incubation period of approximately 4–6 weeks has elapsed. Immunoblot is carried out to exclude false-positive reactions (cf. 3.1.4 'Detection Methods').

3.2.3.2 Direct Detection for *Borrelia*
If an infection is suspected, detection is best carried out with plasma after enrichment via centrifugation or by means of fine-needle biopsy from the inflamed skin around the tick's stinging site. General donor testing for *Borrelia*, e.g. using PCR, is not required.

3.2.4 Donor Interviews
Donors are partly interviewed on a possible exposure after tick bite. This is of little informational value during the winter months. Other signs of bacterial infection, e.g. fever, are recorded based on the usual exclusion criteria.

3.2.5 Donor Information and Counselling
Comprehensive advice is necessary only if the tick bite has been remembered as having occurred within the most recent 1–2 months. In addition to information on *Borrelia*, this advice should also include other relevant arbobacteria and also arboviruses such as tick-borne meningo-encephalitis virus [91].

4 *Francisella tularensis*

4.1 Current Knowledge about the Pathogen

The genus *Francisella* is part of the sub-class of gammaproteobacteria and the order of Thiotrichalis. It forms a family in its own right: the Francisellaceae which is closely related to the family of the Piscirickettsiaceae, and also represents the next relative of the order of Legionellalis (*Coxiella, Rickettsiella*). The bacterium was isolated by McCoy and Chapin [43] from a dead gopher in Tulare, CA, in 1910. 10 years later, Frances [44] described the disease more accurately as deer-fly fever, and also described the human infection [44]. *Francisella* occurs endemically in the entire northern hemisphere, especially in animals living near or on the ground such as rodents and more than 100 other mammals. The natural reservoir has

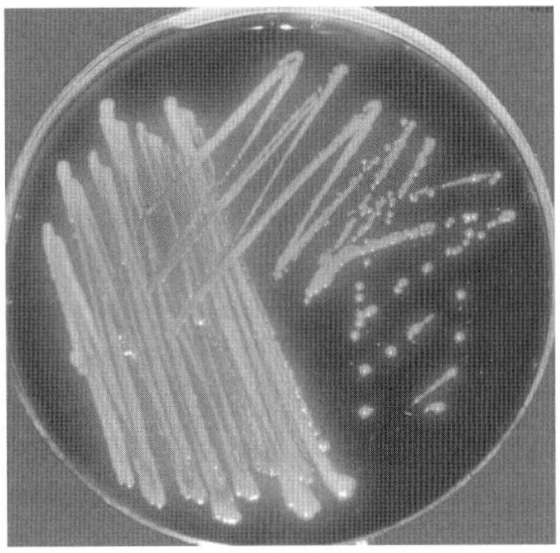

Fig. 2. Cystein-heart-blood agar plate with colonies of *F. tularensis* (PD R. Grunow, Robert Koch-Institute, Berlin, Germany).

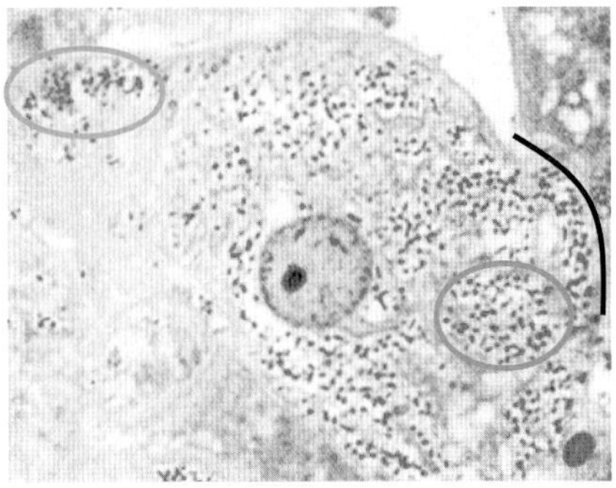

Fig. 3. *Francisella:* Intracellularly accumulated Gram-negative small red shaped bacteria shown within the ovals and restriction to the cytoplasm of one cell as indicated by the black line. Shown is the section of a figure published in ASM News 2003;11:560 [49] previously.

not yet been identified. It is, however, assumed that the pathogen persists in the environment under certain circumstances and in certain animal organisms over a period of months or years.

In addition to transmission by contact with infected animals, laboratory infections also occurred [45]. *Francisella* is transmitted through arthropods as vector, including ticks and midges, as well as by direct contact with infected animals and contaminated environmental materials [46]. Transmission from human to human is unlikely.

There are two species within the *Francisella* genus: *Francisella philomiragia* and *F. tularensis*. The latter is subdivided into 4 sub-species of which *F. tularensis* ssp. tularensis (occurrence in North America) and ssp. holarctica (occurrence in Europe and the entire northern hemisphere) are predominantly human pathogenic [47]. These pathological pictures are related to the entry site of the pathogen and are often characterised by lymph node swelling and skin ulcers. *F. philomiragia* was found in water and soil samples in Texas [48].

F. tularensis ssp. tularensis is considered as hazardous agent potentially usable as biological weapon, and requires culturing under level 3 biosafety laboratory conditions.

4.1.1 Characteristics of the Pathogen

4.1.1.1 Structure

Francisella is a relatively small, faintly stainable, Gram-negative, coccoid, aerobically growing, greyish-white, colony-forming, catalase-positive bacterium. It is immobile, does not form spores and has an electron-transparent lipid-rich capsule which contributes to the virulence of the pathogen.

4.1.1.2 Replication

Francisella grows in the laboratory in sophisticated culture media with blood and a high cystein content, preferably heart-cystein-blood agar, but also chocolate agar or Thayer-Martin agar, which is suitable for gonococci. The culture grows at 37 °C into greyish-white shiny colonies, approximately 3–5 mm in size, in a humid atmosphere with 5–10% CO_2 within 2–5 days. (fig. 2).

10–50 organisms form 1 HID (human infectious dose) after inoculation or inhalation. Approximately 10^8 organisms are required for infection via food. After ingestion, the bacteria replicate intracellularly in lymphoid tissues. Cells of the reticulohistocytic system represent the primary target cells, but hepatocytes are also infected (fig. 3) [49]. Immune response is primarily T lymphocyte-mediated. Antibodies indicate that exposure has taken place. Papule, ulcer and granuloma formation, which may necrotise at a late stage, are characteristic for the disease.

In water, *Francisella* can replicate in amoebae [50]. Infected amoebae are not killed, however, *Francisella* loses some of its virulence in the mouse test by passing into the amoeba.

The bacteria retain their stability under cool and humid conditions for several weeks to months. The pathogen is sensitive to commercial disinfectants and heat treatment. Typically, the bacteria can be killed when treated at temperatures as low as 60 °C for 1 h.

4.1.2 Infection and Infectious Disease

Clinical manifestation essentially depends on the number of inoculated bacteria, their virulence and the host's immune response. The spectrum of disease varies from asymptomatic infection over severe sepsis to death. The incubation period is 3–5 days on average, and ranges from 1–21 days. The infection can be accompanied by sudden occurrence of fever, chills, headache, fatigue, cough, myalgia, breathing trouble and diarrhoea. The fever rises above 39 °C and persists for a few days. Activation of the MglA-regulated genes during growth in the macrophages plays an important part for virulence and pathogenicity [51]. As a rule, the disease can be well treated with an appropriate antibiotic. Depending on the type of pathogen, the lethality rate is as high as 30% or higher in untreated cases [52].

The ulceroglandular form with the typical swelling of the regional lymph nodes develops after inoculation of the pathogen via arthropods or direct contact with contaminated animals, carcass, excrements or other environmental materials. All signs of inflammation accompany the main ulcer, the edge of which hardens. Necrosis in the lymph node may suppurate and

break through towards the interior or the exterior. Super-infections with other bacteria are not unusual.
The oculoglandular form occurs relatively seldom and is usually caused by smear infection. In rare cases, contaminated dusts or aerosols may be the cause.
Oropharyngeal tularaemia manifests itself after oral ingestion of *Francisella*-contaminated food or water. In addition to general symptoms, an almost exclusively one-sided cervical lymph node swelling is characteristic of the disease.
Respiratory tularaemia occurs after inhalation of contaminated dusts and aerosols, usually during farming activities and presents the most severe clinical outcome of tularaemia. In addition to general symptoms, it can manifest itself as a pneumonia-like disease with cough, chest pain and increased respiratory rate. *F. tularensis* can replicate directly in the alveolar epithelial cells after inhalation [53]. Secondary pneumonia after haematogenic spread of the pathogen is also possible. If the pneumonia persists for longer periods, granuloma formation in the X-ray picture can resemble that of tuberculosis.
The term 'typhoid tularaemia' was applied in the past if no typical external signs of tularaemia were visible. Today, this term should only be used in certain circumstances if the route of infection cannot be detected.
Skin erythema occurs in a third of the *Francisella*-infected population 2–3 weeks following infection. This is a manifestation of the bacterial spread and incipient immune response. Absceding and liquefying lymph nodes occur even if the acute signs of illness have subsided.

4.1.3 Epidemiology
F. tularensis has its geographical distribution in the entire northern hemisphere. Persons with a particularly high risk include hunters, farmers, foresters and other groups exposed to outdoor activities for professional or leisure reasons. Among animals, rodents are the preferred reservoir for *Francisella*, but the pathogen also occurs in other mammals and birds. Besides direct contact, arthropods also play an essential part as vectors in the transmission to humans. A prevalence of 0.1–2% has been described for European ticks [54]. Thus, 2% of the ticks in endemic areas are infected with *Francisella* in the Czech Republic and in Austria [55]. Transmission occurs by tick bite of the *Ixodes, Dermatocentor, Amblyomma* species as well as midges of the *Aedes, Culex,* and *Anopheles* species [46]. A third of the 27 hunters and herders in a hare hunt developed *F. tularensis* infection, partly with acute manifestations, in the 'Landkreis' (rural district) of Darmstadt-Dieburg [56] in Hesse, Germany, in 2005 [56].
The occurrence of *Francisella* in freshwater amoebae and the possibility of spreading in water are addressed in Section 4.1.1.2.

4.1.4 Detection Methods

4.1.4.1 Antibodies
Approximately 2 weeks after the occurrence of the clinical symptoms, IgG, IgA, and IgM antibodies can be detected simultaneously. The antibodies thus formed persist for more than 10 years. Available rapid tests include tube or plate agglutination tests the sensitivity of which does not exceed 100% [57]. ELISA and Western Blot assays are used as screening and confirmation tests. These tests are highly sensitive and specific for the holarctica and tularensis subspecies. However, they are currently not yet commercially available and must be adapted to European or North American *Francisella* strains, depending on the requirements [58, 59].

4.1.4.2 Culturing in Medium
F. tularensis does not grow in standard bouillon such as Luria Bertani (LB). The bacterium grows into colonies on blood culture medium enriched with cystein within approximately 48 h at 37 °C under aerobic conditions with 5–10% CO_2. For clinical samples, culturing is best carried out by using smears of skin ulcers or blood. Targeted culturing requires laboratories with biosafety level 3 (in Germany, however, the holarctica subspecies is classified as a pathogen of biohazard level 2). Accompanying flora suppresses the growth of *Francisella*. Suitable mixtures of antibiotics for the shielding of cultures, especially those from environmental samples, are currently being developed. Environmental samples should first be concentrated using 0.45 or 0.22 μm filters, followed by cultivation of the filtered material.

4.1.4.3 Animal Experiment
Another way of culturing is the inoculation of the mouse with material to be tested. *F. tularensis* will grow in the mouse within one week.

4.1.4.4 NAT
Several commercial PCR tests for the detection of *F. tularensis* identify the genomic region of *Francisella* outer membrane protein fopA [60] or the 17-kDa lipoprotein. Differentiation of the subspecies is in most cases successfully carried out using RD1-PCR [62]. PCR is more sensitive than culturing. A TaqMan method for the detection of the bacterium in mammals and vectors has been described [63], and so have a number of other molecular methods for typing *Francisella*.

4.2 Blood and Plasma Donors

4.2.1 Prevalence and Incidence in Donor Populations
In Germany, no transmission of *F. tularensis* via blood has been described to date. A report on the transmission of *F. tularensis* via a kidney transplant is available from Saint Louis, MO, USA. In this report, the infection in the recipient was suc-

cessfully treated with antibiotics following the diagnosis in the donor [64].

4.2.2 Definition of Exclusion Criteria
The general exclusion criteria for donors apply to donors with signs of infection. The main cause of contracting *Francisella* infection in Germany is an injury during gutting of infected hares or the consumption of contaminated meat from hare [56].

4.2.3 Donor Testing and Significance
Because of the epidemiological situation with very low infection numbers and without any known transmission of *F. tularensis* via blood in Germany, testing is currently not required.

Table 2. *Rickettsia* with significance for Europe

Rickettsia	Vector	Disease
R. akari	midge	rickettsial pox
R. conorii	tick	boutonneuse fever, tick bite fever
R. helvetica	tick	spotted fever with slowly healing papules
R. slovaca	tick	spotted fever with slowly healing papules
R. felis	cat flea	cat flea spotted fever (except for humans)
R. prowazekii	louse	epidemic spotted fever, Brill-Zinsser disease – which occurs years after infection, cross-reaction with Proteus OX19 (Weil Felix reaction). The louse dies of the R. infection, louse faeces are infectious.
R. sibirica	louse, tick	spotted fever with slowly healing papules
R. typhi	flea	murine spotted fever; 'Fleckfieber'
R. rickettsii	tick	Rocky Mountains spotted Fieber (only North America – patient's travel history)

5 *Rickettsia*

5.1 Current Knowledge about the Pathogen

Rickettsia is a small Gram-negative obligate intracellular parasite found in mammals, belonging to the alpha proteobacteria species. From the family of *Rickettsia*, the species *Ehrlichia*, *Anaplasma*, and *Orienta* (*Orienta tsutsugamushi*) have been separated based on genetic analyses. The various different *Rickettsia* types are partly categorised into the spotted fever group (SFG – *Rickettsia africa, Rickettsia conori, Rickettsia sibirica, Rickettsia slovaca, R. rickettsii, Rickettsia honei* and *Rickettsia japonica*) and the typhoid group (TG – *Rickettsia typhi* and *R. prowazekii*). This classification has not yet been internationally recognised (table 2).

5.1.1 Characteristics of the Pathogen

5.1.1.1 Structure
Rickettsia is a genus of Gram-negative bacteria that presents as rods of 0.4 to approximately 1.5 µm in length. *Rickettsia* is faintly stainable and not easily visible if Gram staining is applied so that the preferred method is acridine orange staining. The genome is very small, with 1.1–1.6 Mbp. The cell wall contains lipopolysaccharides, peptidoglycans and the outer membrane protein P (Omp P), a small surface protein with approximately 135 kDa, and a 17 kDa lipoprotein [65]. The proteins Omp A and Omp B are only intermittently expressed on the surface during maturation of the bacteria. The lipopolysaccharides of the different *Rickettsia* lead to immunological cross-reaction. *Rickettsia* carry a carbohydrate layer on their surface. They are freely motile within the mammalian cell. In the vector, *Rickettsia* bacteria are transmitted transovarially so that, if they are present in large quantities and replicate strongly, horizontal transmission to the infected mammal is also possible [66].

5.1.1.2 Replication
Rickettsia replicates in cells of the vector and in great numbers of cells of the infected mammal. *Rickettsia* can be cultured and replicated on Vero, HEL and L929 cells.

5.1.2 Infection and Infectious Disease
Rickettsia bacteria are spread via the lymph and blood pathways following inoculation. They adhere to the surface of endothelial and other cells via the proteins Omp A and Omp B. They are phagocytised, escape lysis in the phagosome and move into the cell core. There, they replicate by longitudinal division, are moved to cell surface along the actin skeleton and then released. Cell-to-cell transmission, e.g. in the skin and the lungs, is possible. The infected cell dies after a few days so that bleeding may result after endothelial cell infection. Whether the disease is overcome depends on rapid availability of cytotoxic CD8+ T lymphocytes from the host.
In addition to the skin and the vascular system, manifestation sites of a *Rickettsia* infection include interstitial pneumonia, interstitial myocarditis and perivascular haemorrhage in the brain, gastrointestinal duct and kidney.
The incubation period is 2–14 days, on average 7 days. The body temperature rises above 39 °C.
In case of an *R. conori* infection, clinical outcome is usually mild. The course of the disease of this bacterium is similar to spotted fever. The bacterium occurs in South-East Europe, Africa, the Middle East up to Central Asia. The incubation period is 5–7 days. Clinical signs that stand out the most include swollen lymph nodes with a tendency to superficial haemorrhage at the inoculation site. In the body, the bacterium is usually spread via the blood pathways. The endothelial cells are massively infected. Deaths may occur.
The incubation period of *R. akari* is 10–17 days. The bacterium occurs in North America and Central Europe. In case of *R. akari*, one singular papule per inoculation is formed per bite

from which a vesicle develops which droops centrally, bleeds inward and forms a scab. Regional lymph nodes are swollen. The disease is described as *Rickettsia* pox.

R. prowazekii is the pathogen of the endemic spotted fever (typhus), which has a world-wide distribution. Symptoms include spotted rash and fever which persists 8–10 days and can continue at a level of up to 40 °C. The incubation period is 7–14 days. Initially severe headache and limb pain and the skin exanthema as from day 4–7 are typical symptoms. Depending on the nutritional situation of the infected individual, the death rate can be high (Napoleon army: more than 100,000 deaths). The patient often does not recover entirely. Relapses will then occur frequently, the so-called Brill-Zinsser disease (relapsing disease first described by Nathan Brill in New York in 1898 [67]). The epidemiological connection was established by Hans Zinsser in 1933 [68].

5.1.3 Epidemiology

R. akari and *R. prowazekii* occur world-wide. Transmission depends on the spreading of the vectors and the hygienic conditions. The concerned vector regions remain infectious for decades due to transovarial transmission since agricultural animals are also affected [69]. Wild-animal populations are only partly infected.

5.1.4 Detection Methods

5.1.4.1 Culturing in Media

If there is a history of the exposure and clinical symptoms, *Rickettsia* detection should be performed as early as possible during the infection phase by drawing heparin blood and transferring it onto culture cells. Approximately 0.5 ml heparin blood or extracts of tissue samples are transferred to Vero, L929, HEL, or MRC5 cells before starting treatment of the patient with doxycycline. First growth of the bacteria can be seen after 2–3 days. Detection of *Rickettsia* is carried out by immunofluorescence or immune peroxidase staining. Culturing *Rickettsia* requires a biosafety level 3 laboratory.

5.1.4.2 Antibodies

Indirect immunofluorescence with commercially available *Rickettsia*-infected cells is still the standard. IgM and IgG detection are carried out separately. In addition, antibodies can be detected by latex agglutination (*R. rickettsii*) and ELISA: ELISA assays for the various different *Rickettsia* types, including *Orienta tsutsugamushi*, are commercially available.

When evaluating the results, cross-reactions such as Weil-Felix reaction of *Proteus vulgaris* and *Proteus mirabilis* must also be taken into account. For the detection of an acute infection, it is the increase in titres that is of importance.

5.1.4.3 NAT

PCR is the most reliable method of *Rickettsia* detection. Reliable results are obtained if the gene of the 17 kDa lipoprotein is amplified [70]. The results can be obtained in special laboratories within 6 h [71].

5.2 Blood and Plasma Donors

5.2.1 Prevalence and Incidence in Donor Populations

Routine testing of donors for antibodies or the bacterium is currently not indicated due to the current epidemiological situation. Antibodies against *Rickettsia* have been identified in blood donors in South France (prevalence 5–20% [72]) and Malaysia (prevalence 15% [73]). The *Rickettsia* antibody prevalence depends on the region. Thus, 8% was described for *R. conorii* and 2% for *R. typhi* in North Greece [74], 7% [75] for *R. typhi* in Central Spain and 74% [76] for *R. conorii* in West Spain.

Since *Rickettsia* replicates in endothelial cells, it can be transmitted by blood transfusion in the acute, pre-clinical and relapsing phases. A case of *R. rickettsiae* transmission by blood transfusion was described in 1978, in which the recipient survived after treatment with antibiotics; the donor, however, did not [77].

5.2.2 Definition of Exclusion Criteria

History of tick bites, louse bites, louse infestation, and visits to endemic areas are valid exclusion criteria. The same applies to typical healing papules and scratch marks on the skin.

5.2.3 Donor Testing and Significance

In Germany, donors are not tested for *Rickettsia* antibodies or *Rickettsia* nucleic acid, and this is not required based on the current epidemiological situation.

5.2.4 Donor Interviews

In case of suspected infection, targeted questions on louse infestation and tick bite can contribute to the prevention of *Rickettsia* transmission by blood donation.

5.2.5 Donor Information and Counselling

Advice is indicated, if the donor's history requires this. This advice can also be given by physicians in an external centre with specialised knowledge.

6 *Yersinia pestis*

6.1 Current Knowledge about the Pathogen

Yersinia belongs to the family of Enterobacteriaceae. As psychrophilic bacterium, *Yersinia* is capable of replicating at 4 °C. This ability plays an important part in transfusion medicine. Especially in the case of *Yersinia enterocolitica*, it can lead to a replication if stored in blood reserves [78]. *Yersinia* resides in the soil as well as in animals such as rodents, pigs and birds

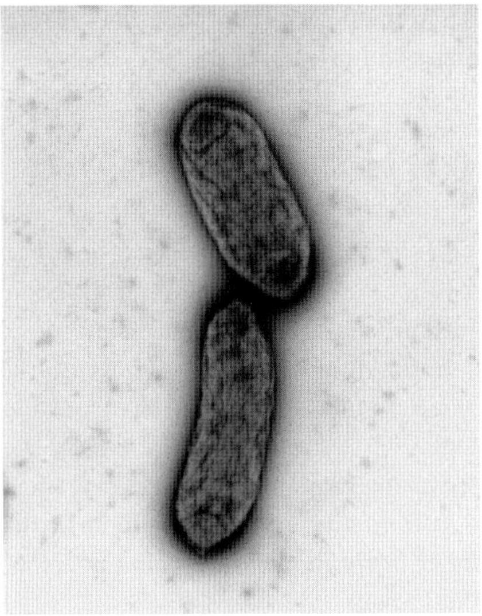

Fig. 4. *Y. pestis*. Photo taken using transmission electron microscopy. The length of the bacterium is approximately 1–2 μm.

[79]. The plague, caused by *Y. pestis*, occurred in three major pandemics in history: Justinian Plague (531–580 AD), the plague of the 14th century, also known as 'The Black Death', and the Hong Kong Plague, which killed more than 100 million people [80].

6.1.1 Characteristics of the Pathogen

6.1.1.1 Structure

Y. pestis is a Gram-negative rod-shaped bacterium with a bipolar staining (giving it a safety-pin appearance, fig. 4). There are three distinct biovars of *Yersinia*: antiqua, mediaevalis, and orientalis. The virulence of *Y. pestis* depends on the presence of different plasmids. The 70 kb virulence plasmid encodes for the expression of the type-III secretion system, which lyses macrophages by contact-dependent injection of effector proteins into these macrophages, and for the V antigen. The 110 kb plasmid encodes for the factor of the anti-phagocytic fraction (Fra 1), and the 9.5 kb plasmid encodes for the temperature-dependent protease (plasminogen activator protein – Pla protease) [80, 81].

6.1.1.2 Replication

Y. pestis grows faster at 28 °C and should be cultivated at 37 °C for at least 48 h. Virulent isolates grow at 37 °C as small colonies compared to avirulent ones. The expression of the genes is controlled on the plasmids depending on the growth temperature, thus influencing the virulence.

6.1.1.3 Extent to which the Bacterium Can Be Inactivated; Stability under Environmental Conditions

For general information, please refer to section 1.1.3. Similarly to other arbobacteria, e.g. *C. burnetii* and *Francisella*, *Y. pestis* is very resistant in the environment. The bacterium grows at temperatures as from 0 °C, and also replicates in coagulated blood. However, the pathogen is sensitive to sun light and can easily be killed by high temperatures and disinfectant.

6.1.2 Infection and Infectious Disease

Pathogenicity is essentially influenced by the structure of the plasmid. This explains why *Y. pestis* strains with different degrees of pathogenicity occur in geographically restricted areas. The immune response in humans is based on antibodies and the rapid formation of cytotoxic T lymphocytes directed against virulence factors encoded by the 70 kb plasmid [82], and directed against Caf1 encoded by the 110 kb plasmid, a protein which acts as a chaperon [83].

6.1.2.1 Rat Flea

In the presence of the 9.5 kb plasmid, *Y. pestis* causes the sucked blood in the flea to coagulate, and *Yersinia* replicates in the coagulum. This leads to an inhibition of the intestinal motility so that the blood is regurgitated at the next sucking action, and thousands of *Yersinia* are injected into the skin of the rat or human.

6.1.2.2 Human – Bubonic Plague

This type of plague is the most common form of manifestation. Fever (38.5–40 °C) and chills suddenly occur within an incubation period of 2–7 days. Painfully swollen lymph nodes develop within few hours, which form part of the regional drainage area at the inoculation site of the rat flea. The size can be up to 10 cm. Affected limbs – the bite usually occurs at the extremities – are spared. Suppurating ulceration of the lymph node can occur. Papules and pustules can occur adjacent to the lymph nodes. There are signs of bacterial metastases. Bacteriaemia is detectable in 80% of the bubonic plague.

6.1.2.3 Septic Plague

If the bacteria cannot be retained in the lymph node, sepsis occurs. The patient rapidly becomes moribund. Primary sepsis without the lymph node swelling phase or without pneumonia might occur. If not treated, sepsis rapidly leads to death the preliminary phase of which is intravascular coagulation leading to peripheral suboptimal blood circulation making the skin appear deep purple, giving this disease its name 'Black Death'.

6.1.2.4 Pneumonic Plague

The lung is affected by inhalation of the pathogen or haematogenic dissemination of *Y. pestis*. Symptoms include tachypnoea, dyspnoea, cough and bloody sputum. The sputum is purulent. *Y. pestis* can be transmitted directly to individuals in the vicinity by its great number of bacteria in the secretion or sputum via smear infection or aerosol. Transmission from human to human, however, occurs very seldom. If left untreated, pneumonic plague leads to death.

6.1.2.5 Treatment of *Y. pestis*

Streptomycin or gentamycin is the treatment of choice. In addition, doxycycline and ciprofloxacine are also effective. Chloramphenicol is effective for the treatment of plague meningitis. Resistant *Y. pestis* strains are very rare in endemic regions.

6.1.3 Epidemiology

Plague is a typical zoonosis, transmitted by vector bite. Its enzootic occurrence currently includes many natural endemic areas in many countries in Africa, the two Americas and Asia. Outbreaks occur annually with 100–1,000 affected individuals. Up to now, endemic areas for *Y. pestis* can be found in the south of Africa including Madagascar, Southern Russia to India, Mongolia, China, Indonesia, the west of North America, and the centre of South America.

Essentially, the hosts are rats (*Rattus rattus, Rattus norwegicus*), and the essential carrier is the rat flea (*Xenopsylla cheopis*). Other animal hosts include the gopher, the rabbit, the field mouse, and more seldom the dromedary. Other epidemiologically relevant vectors beside the flea are not known.

6.1.4 Detection Methods

In case of suspected *Y. pestis* infection, bacteriologic diagnostics must be performed in a biosafety level 3 laboratory.

6.1.4.1 Antibodies

Antibodies are detectable 1–2 weeks after occurrence of the symptoms. In approximately 5% of all infected individuals, no antibodies are detectable. ELISA assays have been developed for IgM and IgG.

6.1.4.2 Culturing in Media

Y. pestis grows in most culture media, as mentioned above, better at 28 °C than at 37 °C. Suitable culture media are McConkey blood and modified CIN (Cefsulodin Irgasan Novobiocin) agar in aerobic conditions. The small translucent colonies are detectable after 24–48 h depending on the temperature. Differentiation is carried out via biochemically detected enzyme performance and motility of *Y. pestis*, as well as via molecular biology and immunology methods.

6.1.4.3 NAT

Several methods have been published on the detection by means of PCR; above all, under the aspect that *Y. pestis* can be used as a biological weapon. An advantage of PCR compared with the tedious biochemical characterisation is that detection is possible directly from the colony material or even the sample, and that the presence of *Y. pestis* can be safely confirmed within approximately 2–3 h. Several real-time PCR assays have been described: Chase et al. [84] has used the chromosomal marker yp48 for the distinction of *Y. pestis* from other *Yersinia* types. Other tests are based on the detection of *Y. pestis*-specific plasmids [85, 86].

According to Section 6 of the German Infektionsschutzgesetz (Infection Protection Act), the detection of *Y. pestis*, clinically suspected *Y. pestis* infection, and the disease and death due to the pathogen are notifiable.

6.2 Blood and Plasma Donors

6.2.1 Prevalence and Incidence in Donor Populations

Since *Y. pestis* only occurs in endemic areas and outside Germany, no figures have been collected for Germany. Patients infected with *Y. pestis* show signs of acute inflammation and are therefore generally excluded from blood donation.

6.2.2 Definition of Exclusion Criteria

The general criteria for donors with signs of infection apply. Lymph node swelling and signs of fever are initial symptoms of the infection. The deferral for donors returning from tropical areas only applies to part of the individuals returning from endemic areas. Interviews on the donor history may help clarify an indication to an infection.

6.2.3 Donor Testing and Significance

Based on the epidemiologic situation, no infections due to blood donation have become known in the past few decades. Thus, testing for *Y. pestis* is currently not required.

7 Facts about all Arbobacteria

Arbobacteria can retain their ability to replicate in the soil or in water in fresh water amoebae for months, thus showing great resistance to the environment. Analogous with other non-spore formers, heating to 65–70 °C for 10 min and chemical treatment with 1% phenol, 5% hydrogen peroxide, 5% chloroform, 0.5% hypochlorite, and 5% formaldehyde for 10–30 min are considered as effective for inactivation. Disinfecting with 70% ethanol for 1 min also inactivates arbobacteria.

7.1 Recipients

7.1.1 Prevalence and Incidence of Blood-Associated Infections and Infectious Diseases in Recipient Populations

Few data are available on the prevalence and incidence in recipients in Germany. Regionally different immunity, above all, exists for infections with *Borrelia* which depends on the tick occurrence, the infection of ticks with *Borrelia*, and the leisure time behaviour and profession of the recipient. For *Anaplasma, Ehrlichia, Bartonella, Francisella* and *Rickettsia*, antibody prevalences are in the low percentile. Exposure to *Y. pestis* is not assumed for persons living in Germany.

The following antibody prevalences are assumed according to a study by Raoult [1] in France:

- *Bartonella:* 0.1–0.001%,
- *Borrelia:* 1–0.01%,
- *Francisella:* 0.1–0.001%,
- *R. prowazekii:* up to 35% infection rate in homeless individuals,

- R. typhi: 0.001%,
- Ehrlichia: 0.01% in the USA [10].

7.1.2 Immune Status (Resistance, Existing Immunity, Immune Response, Age, Exogenous Factors)

The defence situation depends on the general state of the infected individual, his/her existing immunity, immunoreactivity, age and exogenous factors. The essential factor causing chronic outcome of the infection by arbobacteria results from the primarily intracellular growth of arbobacteria and continued change of the antigenic surface profile. Infectiousness of blood cannot be removed from blood entirely by leukocyte depletion since the bacteria are also present extracellularly.
Small amounts of free bacteria are removed by unspecific defence mechanisms, such as complement lysis, opsonisation and lipopolysaccharide-directed phagocytosis, as well as other mechanisms of the congenital immune defences. Since the defence mechanisms decrease with age, in over 60-year-olds chronic outcome and/or relapse of the infection must be expected after transmission of the infection (cf. Brill-Zinsser disease under *R. prowazekii*). Possible complications such as abscess formation, endocarditis, myocarditis, encephalitis and immunoreactive arthritis also occur more frequently in older individuals.
After transfusion of a bacterially contaminated blood reserve, first antibodies are detectable within 2–3 weeks as measurable immune response and the pathogen can be detected via NAT, at least in specialised laboratories, within 2–3 weeks at the earliest (cf. 6.1.4.3). Fulminant and rapidly deadly outcomes have been described for *Bartonella, Francisella* and *Rickettsia* infections in case of immune deficiency, especially caused by HIV [1]. For patients without immune deficiency diseases, primary major symptoms of arbobacteria transmission include high, partly relapsing fever, particularly induced by the released lipopolysaccharide (endotoxin). Fever does not necessarily occur in the case of an immune deficiency, nor does the typical lymph node swelling [87].
The further outcome for the infected receiver is basically determined by rapidly induced antibiotic treatment, as shown e.g. for *R. rickettsii* transmission by blood transfusion [77].

7.1.2.1 Vaccination

A vaccine has been developed only against *B. burgdorferi*, and has been used in approximately 450,000 individuals in the USA [88]. This vaccine has been withdrawn from the market because of the occurrence of unclarified arthritis which has been in questionable causal relationship with the vaccination. No vaccine has been available so far for humans against infection with the other arbobacteria. In animals, too, vaccine development is difficult. Thus, the vaccination has not been generally used against *Afipia (Bartonella) felis* in cats or against *C. burnetii* in sheep.
Vaccines against *R. rickettsii* were developed and also tested in Germany before and during World War II, above all for military interests, but could not reach pre-marketing stage due to inadequate protectiveness and considerable adverse effects [1] so that no vaccine is available today. Proteins influencing pathogenicity in *F. tularensis* infections have been successful in early vaccination attempts [89]. A live vaccine of *F. tularensis* with a deleted protein, which influences purin metabolism, creates immunity in mice protecting them from a deadly dose of the wild-type bacterium [90]. Partial immunity against *Y. pestis* with a vaccine consisting of Cafl protein can be created in mice [83].

7.1.3 Severity and Course of the Disease

About two thirds of the infections with arbobacteria have an asymptomatic and self-limiting outcome in immunocompetent individuals (see above). As the example of *R. rickettsii* shows, in case of clinical manifestation, a mild outcome and survival of the recipient is possible in case of early treatment (4th day), whereas the donor died without treatment [77]. Chronic arbobacteria infections manifest themselves with the usual signs of inflammation caused by bacterial toxins such as irregular febrile episodes, night sweat, exhaustion, fatigue, lymphatic adenopathy, arthritis of the small and large joints up to perivasculitis, endocarditis, myocarditis and encephalitis. Tick, louse and flea bites cannot always be identified from the patient's history. Since treatment is effective and without any major adverse effect, rapid antibiotic treatment should be started in case of suspected infection, even without specific pathogen identification; rapid treatment influences the survival rate, particularly in case of *Y. pestis* infection.

7.1.4 Therapy and Prophylaxis

7.1.4.1 Therapy

In case of unknown arbobacterium, doxycycline is the treatment of choice. Chloramphenicol, ampicilline, and cephalosporine are also very effective. As a rule, quinolone is effective in high dosages (750 mg twice daily for 5–7 days). Quinolone is only partly effective against *Rickettsia*. For *Yersinia*, a combination therapy with doxycycline and gentamicine should currently be the most effective one.
Since most pathogens, except for *Y. pestis*, grow intracellularly, treatment should continue for 2–3 weeks. Administration for a longer period is recommended if the nervous system is involved. Repeated infection, e.g. with *Borrelia*, will create partial immunity so that the *Borrelia* pathogens can be inactivated or eliminated via the immune system in case of re-infection without the occurrence of clinical symptoms.

7.1.4.2 Prophylaxis

In line with the main route of transmission, exposure to ticks and other vectors listed in Section 1.1 should be avoided in order to prevent infection. The pathogen can be transmitted by direct contact with *Bartonella, Coxiella, Francisella* and

Yersinia. Contaminations with these bacteria have also occurred in the laboratory.

7.1.5 Transmissibility

In principle, arbobacteria can be transmitted by a vector (for an exception, see 7.1.4.2). All arbobacteria at least temporarily infect endothelial cells, macrophages and neutrophil granulocytes, and can cause temporary bacteriaemia. They are transmissible via blood and/or erythrocyte and thrombocyte concentrates, especially in the acute initial stage of the infection. However, infections by arbobacteria have so far not been reported in Germany.

7. 1.6 Frequency of Administration, Type and Amount of Blood Products

Up to now, no transmission of arbobacteria via the blood which would be possible at the acute and the chronic stage of the infection has become known in Germany. Since the disease leads to signs of inflammation and to donor exclusion in compliance with the general guidelines, a large number of undiagnosed and unregistered transmissions should not be expected.

Transmission of arbobacteria via fresh frozen plasma is theoretically possible. Transmission by plasma derivatives can be excluded thanks to the manufacturing process since the bacteria are eliminated and inactivated entirely. Both heat inactivation and detergent treatment of plasma components will lead to loss of infectivity of the arbobacteria.

7.2 Blood Products

7. 2.1 Infectious Load of the Starting Material and Test Methods

Burden of blood or plasma with arbobacteria is unknown, but is to be considered as extremely low in Germany for reasons of infection epidemiology. For bacteria transmissible only by ticks, an accumulation of infections, if any, should only be seasonal; however, this has so far not been observed.

Since all arbobacteria also grow intracellularly and occur extracellulary, they cannot be removed from blood or cell-containing blood components.

7.2.2 Methods for Removal and Inactivation of the Infectious Agent

7.2.2.1 Separation

Arbobacteria cannot be removed from blood or cell-containing blood components. Leukocyte depletion can lead to pathogen reduction, e.g. for *Ehrlichia, Francisella* or *Rickettsia*, but cannot lead to complete removal.

In principle, bacteria can be removed from plasma by high revolution centrifugation or filtration over 0.22 μm filters. Neither method is feasible for fresh frozen plasma. Small bacteria such as *Coxiella, Rickettsia* and other arbobacteria types, but not *Borrelia* and *Yersinia*, can also penetrate filters of that pore size [2].

7.2.2.2 Inactivation

Arbobacteria can be inactivated by heat treatment >65 °C for 10 h or by pasteurising, e.g. at 60 °C for 10 h. For Gram-negative bacteria, lipopolysaccharide is released from the cell wall by heat treatment. If administered i.v., lipopolysaccharide can lead to febrile reaction up to endotoxin shock.

In thrombocyte concentrates, arbobacteria can be inactivated by treatment with psoralen or similar substances.

7.2.3 Feasibility and Validation of Procedures for Removal/ Inactivation of the Infectious Agent

Arbobacteria can partly be replicated in cell culture to achieve quantities which allow spiking of blood or plasma. For *F. tularensis* ssp. tularensis, biosafety level 3 is required in compliance with the regulations for biological substances (Biostoff-Verordnung), safety level 2 is required for *Anaplasma, Bartonella, Borrellia* and *Ehrlichia*.

Validation of the procedures for epidemiological reasons is currently not necessary, especially since no arbobacteria infection by blood transmission has become known.

7.3 Assessment

Arbobacteria are pathogens which grow intracellularly and can replicate also in endothelial cells and macrophages or granulocytes, and are transmissible by blood. If transmitted, the pathogens can cause severe and even deadly infections. If the course is chronic, the disease can be consuming with organ function impairment.

Prevalence of arbobacteria infections is very low in Germany, except for *B. burgdorferi, B afzelii* and *B. garinii* infections, which can reach a prevalence of 10–30%, particularly in endemic areas.

The generally low risk of transmission of arbobacteria can be further prevented if donors with reduced hygienic status are excluded from donation. Acutely and chronically infected blood donors are recorded by their clinical symptoms and by general donor exclusion criteria, and the exclusion criteria have proved to be effective.

The low significance of arbobacteria transmission is proved by the fact that no transfusion-related transmission has been reported in Germany in the past 30 years. Arbobacteria have currently no significance for the safety of blood products and plasma derivatives in Germany.

This paper was completed on March 19, 2007 and approved by the German Advisory Committee Blood (Arbeitskreis Blut) on May 30, 2007. It was compiled by the members of the subgroup 'Assessment of Pathogens Transmissible by Blood' of the German Advisory Committee Blood (Arbeitskreis Blut):

Prof. Dr. Lutz Gürtler
Dr. Johannes Blümel
Prof. Dr. Reinhard Burger
Dr. Christian Drosten
Dr. Albrecht Gröner
Dr. Margarethe Heiden
Dr. Walter Hitzler
Prof. Dr. Dr. Bernd Jansen
Dr. Horst Klamm
Prof. Dr. Wolf-Dieter Ludwig
Dr. Thomas Montag-Lessing
Dr. Ruth Offergeld
Prof. Dr. Georg Pauli
Prof. Dr. Rainer Seitz
Dr. Uwe Schlenkrich
Dr. Volkmar Schottstedt
Dr. Hannelore Willkommen.

References

1 Raoult D: Introduction to rickettsiosis and ehrlichiosis; in Mandell GL, Bennett JE, Dolin R (eds): Principles and Practice of Infectious Diseases, 6th ed. Philadelphia, Elsevier, 2005, pp 2284–2287.

2 Arbeitskreis Blut, Untergruppe 'Bewertung Blutassoziierter Krankheitserreger': *Coxiella burnetii* – Erreger des Q- (query) Fiebers. Bundesgesundheitsbl Gesundheitsforsch Gesundheitsschutz 2005; 48:814–821.

3 Houhamdi L, Lepidi H, Drancourt M, Raoult D: Experimental model to evaluate the human body louse as a vector of plague. J Infect Dis 2006;194: 1589–1596.

4 Maeda K, Markowitz N, Hawley RC, Ristic M, Cox D, McDade JE: Human infection with *Ehrlichia canis*, a leukocytic *Rickettsia*. N Engl J Med 1987; 316:853–856.

5 Walker DH, Dumler JS: *Ehrlichia chaffeensis* (human monocytotropic ehrlichiosis), *Anaplasma phagocytophilum* (human granulocytotropic anaplasmosis) and other Ehrlichiae; in Mandell GL, Bennett JE, Dolin R (eds): Principles and Practice of Infectious Diseases, 6th ed. Philadelphia, Elsevier, 2005, pp 2310–2318.

6 Hildebrandt A, Schmidt KH, Wilske B, Dorn W, Straube E, Fingerle V: Prevalence of four species of *Borrelia burgdorferi* sensu lato and coinfection with *Anaplasma phagocytophila* in *Ixodes ricinus* ticks in central Germany. Eur J Clin Microbiol Infect Dis 2003;22:364–367.

7 Wielinga PR, Gaasenbeek C, Fonville M, Boer AD, Vries AD, Dimmers W, Jagers GAO, Schouls LM, Borgsteede F, Giessen JWBVD: Longitudinal analysis of tick densities and *Borrelia, Anaplasma* and *Ehrlichia* infections of *Ixodes ricinus* ticks in different habitat areas in The Netherlands. Appl Envrion Microbiol 2006;72:7594–7601.

8 Standaert SM, Yu T, Scott MA, Childs JE, Paddock CD, Singleton NJ, Blaser MJ: Primary isolation of *Ehrlichia chaffeensis* from patients with febrile illness: clinical and molecular characteristics. J Infect Dis 2000;181:1082–1088.

9 Anderson BE, Sumner JW, Dawson JE, Tzianabos T, Greene CR, Olson JG, Fishbein DB, Olsen-Rasmussen M, Hollowau BP, George EH, Azad AF: Detection of the etiologic agent of human ehrlichiosis by polymerase chain reaction. J Clin Microbiol 1992;30:775–780.

10 Standaert SM, Dawson JE, Schaffner W, Childs JE, Biggie KL, Singleton J, Gerhardt RR, Knight ML, Hutcheson RH: Ehrlichiosis in a golf oriented retirement community. N Engl J Med 1995;333: 420–425.

11 Brouqui P, Lecam C, Olson J, Raoult D: Serologicc diagnosis of human monocytic ehrlichiosis by immunoblot analysis. Clin Diag Lab Immunol 1994; 1:645–649.

12 Dreher UM, Fuente JDL, Hofmann-Lehmann R, Meli ML, Pusterla N, Kocan KM, Woldehiwet Z, Braun U, Regula G, Staerk KDC, Lutz H: Serologic cross-rectivity between *Anaplasma marginale* and *Anaplasma phagocytophilum*. Clin Diag Lab Immunol 2005;12:1177–1183.

13 Trofe J, Reddy KS, Stratta RJ, Flax SD, Somerville KT, Alloway RR, Egidi MF, Shokouh-Amiri MH, Gaber AO: Human granulocytic ehrlichiosis in pancreas transplant recipients. Transpl Infect Dis 2001; 3:34–39.

14 Leiby DA, Chung AP, Cable RG, Trouern-Trend J, McCullough J, Homer MJ, Reynolds LD, Houghton RL, Lodes MJ, Persing DH: () Relationship between tick bites and the seroprevalence of *Babesia microti* and *Anaplasma phagocytophila* (previously *Ehrlichia* sp) in blood donors. Transfusion 2002; 42:1585–1591.

15 Fingerle V, Goodman JL, Johnson RC, Kurtti TJ, Munderloh UG, Wilske B: Human granulocytic ehrlichiosis in Southern Germany; increased seroprevalence in high risk groups. J Clin Microbiol 1997;35:3244–3247.

16 Fingerle V, Munderloh UG, Liegl G, Wilske B: Coexsistence of *Ehrlichia* of the phagocytophila group with *Borrelia burgdorferi* in *Ixodes ricinus* from Southern Germany. Med Microbiol Immuno 1999; 188:145–149.

17 Del Prete R, Fumarola D, Fumarola L, Basile V, Mosca A, Miragliotta G: Prevalence of antibodies to *Bartonella henselae* in patients with suspected cat scratch disease (CSD) in Italy. Eur J Epidemiol 1999;15:583–587.

18 McGill S, Wesslen L, Hjelm E, Holmberg M, Rolf C, Friman G: Serological and epidemiological analysis of the prevalence of B spp antibodies in Swedish elite orienteers 1992–93. Scand J Infect Dis 2001;33:423–428.

19 Mallqui V, Speelmon EC, Verastegui M, Maguina-Vargas C, Pinell-Salles P, Lavarello R, Delgado J, Kosek M, Romero S, Arana Y, Gilman RH: Sonicated diagnostic immunoblot for bartonellosis. Clin Diagn Lab Immunol 2000;7:1–5.

20 Handley SA, Regnery RL: Differentiation of pathogenic *Bartonella* species by infrequent restriction site PCR. J Clin Microbiol 2000;38:3010–3015.

21 Kordick DL, Breitschwerdt EB: Relapsing bacteriemia after blood transfusion of *Bartonella henselae* to cats. Am J Vet Res 1997;58:492–497.

22 Steere AC, Malawista SE, Snydman DR, Shope RE, Andiman WA, Ross MR, Steele FM: Lyme arthritis: An epidemic of oligoarticular arthritis in children and adults in three Connecticut communities. Arthritis Rheum 1977;20:7–17.

23 Bannwarth A: Chronische lymphozytäre Menigitis, entzündliche Polyneuritis und 'Rheumatismus'. Arch Psychiatr Nervenkrankh 1941;111:284–376.

24 Herxheimer K, Hartmann K: Über Acrodermatitis chronica atrophicans. Arch Dermatol Syph 1902;61: 57–76,255–300

25 Afzelius A: Bericht der Verhandlungen der Dermatologischen Gesellschaft zu Stockholm am 16. Dezember 1909. Arch Dermatol Syph 1910;101:405.

26 Fraser CM, Casjens S, Huang WM, Sutton GG, Clayton R, Lathigra R, White O, Ketchum KA, Dodson R, Hickey EK, Gwinn M, Dougherty B, Tomb JF, Fleischmann RD, Richardson D, Peterson J, Kerlavage AR, Quackenbush J, Salzberg S, Hanson M, van Vugt R, Palmer N, Adams MD, Gocayne J, Weidman J, Utterback T, Watthey L, McDonald L, Artiach P, Bowman C, Garland S, Fuji C, Cotton MD, Horst K, Roberts K, Hatch B, Smith HO, Venter JC: Genomic sequence of a Lyme disease spirochete, *Borrelia burgdorferi*. Nature 1997; 390:580–586.

27 Schulte-Spechtel U, Lehnert G, Liegl G, Fingerle V, Heimerl C, Johnson BJB, Wilske B: Significant improvement of the recombinant *Borrelia*-specific immunoglobulin G immunoblot test by addition of VlsE and a DbpA homologue derived from *Borrelia garinii* for diagnosis of early neuroborreliosis. J Clin Microbiol 2003;41:1299–1303.

28 Ramamoorthi N, Narasimhan S, Pal U,Bao F, Yang XF, Fish D, Anguita J, Norgard MV, Kantor FS, Anderson JF, Koski RA, Fikrig E: The Lyme disease agent exploits a tick protein to infect the mammalian host. Nature 2005;436:573–577.

29 Wilske B, Schriefer ME: () *Borrelia*; in Murray PR, Baron EJ, Jorgensen JH, Pfaller MA, Yolken RH (eds): Manual of Clinical Micriobiology, 8th ed. Washington, DC, ASM Press, 2003, pp 937–954.

30 Steere AC: Lyme disease. N Engl J Med 1989; 321:586–596.

31 Wilske B, Münchhoff P, Schierz G, Preac-Mursic V, Roggendorf M, Zoulek G: Zur Epidemiologie der *Borrelia burgdorferi*-Infektion. Münch Med Wochenschr 1985;127:171–172.

32 Tomao P, Ciceroni L, Ovidio MCD, Rosa MD, Vonesch N, Iavicoli S, Signorini S, Ciarocchi S, Ciufolini MG, Fiorentini C, Papaleo B: Prevalence and incidence of antibodies to *Borrelia burgdorferi* and to tick-borne encephalitis virus in agricultural and forestry workers from Tuscany, Italy. Eur J Clin Microbiol Infect 2005;24:457–463.

33 Lledo L, Gegundez MI, Saz JV, Beltran M: Screening of the prevalence of antibodies to *Borrelia burgdorferi* in Madrid province, Spain. Eur J Epidemiol 2004;19:471–472.
34 Hauser U, Lehnert G, Lobentanzer R, Wilske B: Interpretation criteria for standardized western blots for three European species of *Borrelia burgdorferi* sensu lato. J Clin Microbiol 1997;35:1433–1444.
35 Nocton JJ, Dressler F, Rutledge BJ, Rys PN, Persing DH, Steere AC: Detection of *Borrelia burgdorferi* DNA by polymerase chain reaction in synovial fluid from patients with Lyme arthritis. N Engl J Med 1994;330:229–234.
36 Vasiliu V, Herzer D, Rössler D, Lehnert G, Wilske B: Heterogeneity of *Borrelia burgdorferi* sensu lato demonstrated by an OspA type specific PCR in synovial fluid from patients with Lyme arthritis. Med Microbiol Immunol 1998;187:97–102.
37 Nadal D, Wunderli W, Briner H, Hansen K: Prevalence of antibodies to *Borrelia burgdorferi* in forestry workers and blood donors from the same region in Switzerland. Eur J Clin Microbiol Infect Dis 1989;8:992–995.
38 Bohme M, Schwenecke S,Fuchs E, Wiebecke D, Karch H: Screening of blood donors and recipients for *Borrelia* antibodies: no evidence of *B. burgdorferi* infection transmitted by transfusion. Infusionsther Transfusionsmed 1992;19:204–207.
39 Weiland T, Kühnl P, Laufs R, Heesemann J: Prevalence of *Borrelia burgdorferi* antibodies in Hamburg blood donors; in Kretschmer V, Stangel W, Wiebecke D (Hrsg): Transfusionsmedizin 1991/92. Beitr Infusionsther. Basel, Karger, 1992, vol 30, pp 92–95.
40 Johnson SE, Swaminathan B, Moore P, Broome CV, Parvin M: *Borrelia burgdorferi*: survival in experimentally infected human blood processed for transfusion. J Infect Dis 1990;162:557–559.
41 Nadelman RB, Sherer C, Mack L, Pavia CS, Wormser GP: Survival of *Borrelia burgdorferi* in human blood stored under blood banking conditions. Transfusion 1990;30:298–301.
42 Gerber MA, Shapiro ED, Krause PJ, Cable RG, Badon SJ, Ryan RW: The risk of acquiring Lyme disease or babesiosis from a blood transfusion. J Infect Dis 1994;170:231–234.
43 McCoy GM, Chapin CW: Bacterium tularense the cause of a plaque-like disease of rodents. US Public Health Hosp Bull 1912;53:17–23.
44 Francis E: The occurrence of tularemia in nature as a disease of man. US Public Health Rep 1921; 36:1731–1738.
45 Penn RL: *Francisella tularensis* (Tularemia); in Mandell GL, Bennett JE, Dolin R (eds): Principles and Practice of Infectious Diseases, 6th ed. Philadelphia, Elsevier, 2005, pp 2674–2685.
46 Ellis J, Oyston PC, Green M, Titball RW: Tularemia. Clin Microbiol Rev 2002;15:631–646.
47 Petersen JM, Schriefer ME: Tularemia: emergence/re-emergence. Vet Res 2005;36:455–467.
48 Barns SM, Grow CC, Okinaka RT, Keim P, Kuske CR: Detection of diverse new *Francisella* like bacteria in environmental samples. Appl Environ Micrbiol 2005;71:5494–5500.
49 Titball RW, Sjöstedt A: *Francisella tularensis*: an overview. ASM News 2003;11:558–563.
50 Berdal BP, Mehl R, Meidell NK, Lorentzen-Styr AM, Scheel O: Field investigations of tularemia in Norway. FEMS Immunol Med Microbiol 1996; 13:191–195.
51 Brotcke A, Weiss DS, Kim CC, Chain P, Malfatti S, Garcia E, Monck DM: Identification of MglA-regulated genes reveals novel virulence factors in *Francisella tularensis*. Infect Immun 2006;74:6642–6655.
52 Staples JE, Kubota KA, Chalcraft LG, Mead PS, Petersen JM: Epidemiologic and molecular analysis of human tularemia, United States, 1964–2004. Emerg Infect Dis 2006;12:1113–1118.
53 Hall JD, Craven RR, Fuller JR, Pickless RJ, Kawula TH: *Francisella tularensis* replicates within alveolar type II epithelial cells in vitro and in vivo following inhalation. Infect Immun 2007;75:1034–1039.
54 Gurycova D, Kocianova E, Vyrostekova V, Rehacek J: Prevealence of ticks infected with *Francisella tularensis* in natural foci of tularemia in western Slovakia. Eur J Epidemiol 1995;11:469–474.
55 Hubalek Z, Sixl W, Halouzka J: *Francisella tularensis* in *Dermatocenter reticularis* ticks from the Czech Republic and Austria. Wien Klin Wochenschr 1998; 110:909–910.
56 Robert Koch-Institut: Tularämie: Ausbruch unter Teilnehmern einer Hasen-Treibjagd im Landkreis Darmstadt-Dieburg, 2005. Epidemiol Bull 2005;50: 465–466.
57 Tärnvik A: Nature of protective immunity to *Francisella tularensis*. Rev Infect Dis 1989;11:440–451.
58 Porsch-Ozcurumez M, Kischel N, Priebe H, Splettstosser W, Finke EJ, Grunow R: Comparison of enzyme-linked immunosorbent assay, Western blotting, microagglutination, indirect immunofluorescence assay, and flow cytometry for serological diagnosis of tularemia. Clin Diagn Lab Immunol 2004;11:1008–1015.
59 Bevanger L, Maeland JA, Naess AI: Competitive enzyme immunoassay for antibodies to a 43,000 molecular weight *Francisella tularensis* outer membrane protein for the diagnosis of tularemia. J Clin Microbiol 1989;27:922–926.
60 Fulop M, Leslie D, Titball R: A rapid, highly sensitive method for the detection of *Francisella tularensis* in clinical samples using the polymerase chain reaction. Am J Trop Med Hyg 1996;54:364–366.
61 Grunow RW, Spletstoesser W, McDonald S, Otterbein C, O'Brien T, Morgan C, Aldrich J, Hoffer E, Finke E, Meyer H: Detection of *Francisella tularensis* in biologiocal specimens using a capture enzyme-linked immunosorbent assay, an immunochromatochraphic handheld assay, and a PCR. Clin Diagn Lab Immunol 2000;7:86–90.
62 Broekhuijsen M, Larsson P, Johansson A, Bystrom M, Eriksson U, Larsson E, Prior RG, Sjostedt A, Titball RW, Forsman M: Genome-wide DNA microarray analysis of *Francisella tularensis* strains demonstrates extensive genetic conservation within the species but identifies regions that are unique to the highly virulent *F. tularensis* subsp. tularensis. J Clin Microbiol 2003;41:2924–2931.
63 Higgins JA, Hubalek Z, Halouzka J, Elkins KL, Sjostedt A, Shipley M, Ibrahim MS: Detection of *Francisella tularensis* in infected mammals and vectors using a probe-based polymerase chain reation. Am J Trop Med Hyg 2000;62:310–318.
64 Khoury JA, Bohl DL, Hersh MJ, Argoudelis AC, Brennan DC: Tularemia in a kidney transplant recipient: an unsuspected case and literature review. Am J Kidney Dis 2005;45:926–929.
65 Vishwanath S: Antigenic relationships among the rickettsiae of the spotted fever and typhus group. FEMS Microbiol Lett 1991;81:341–344.
66 McDade JE, Shepard CC, Redus MA, Newhouse VF, Smith JD: Evidence of *Rickettsia prowazekii* infections in the United States. Am J Trop Med Hyg 1980;29:277–284.
67 Brill NE: An acute infectious disease of unknown origin. Am J Med Sci 1910;139:484–502.
68 Zinsser H: Varieties of typhus virus and the epidemiology of the American form of European typhus fever (Brill's disease). Am J Hyg 1934;20: 513–532.
69 Dupont HT, Brouqui P, Faugere B, Raoult D: Prevalence of antibodies to *Coxiella burnetii, Rickettsia conorii*, and *Rickettsai typhi* in seven African countries. Clin Infect Dis 1995;21:1126–1133.
70 Schriefer ME, Sacci JB, Dumler JS, Bullen MG, Azad AF: Identification of a novel rickettsial infection in a patient diagnosed with murine typhus. J Clin Microbiol 1994;32:949–954.
71 Tzianabos T, Anderson BE, McDade JE: Detection of *Rickettsia rickettsii* DNA in clinical specimens by using polymerase chain reaction technology. J Clin Microbiol 1989;27:2866–2868.
72 Raoult D, Toga B, Chaudet H, Chiche-Portiche C: Rickettsial antibody in southern France: antibodies to *Rickettsia conorii* and *Coxiella burnetii* among urban, suburban and semi-rural blood donors. Trans Roy Soc Trop Med Hyg 1987;81:80–81.
73 Tay ST, Kamalanathan M, Rohani MY: Antibody prevalence of *Orienta tsutsugamushi, Rickettsia typhi* and TT118 spotted fever group rickettsiae among Malaysian blood donors and febrile patients in the urban areas. Southeast Asian J Trop Med Public Health 2003;34:165–170.
74 Daniel SA, Manika K, Arvanmdou M, Antoniadis A: Prevalence of *Rickettsia conorii* and *Rickettsia typhi* infections in the population of Northern Greece. Am J Trop Med Hyg 2002;66:76–79.
75 Lledo L, Gegundez MI, Saz JV, Beltran M: Prevalence of antibodies to *Rickettsia typhi* in an area of the center of Spain. Eur J Epidemiol 2001;17: 927–928.
76 Ruiz-Beltran R, Herrero-Herrero JI, Martin-Sanchez AM, Martin-Gonzales JA: Prevalence of antibodies to *Rickettsia conorii, Coxiella burnetii* and *Rickettsia typhi* in Salamanca Province (Spain). Serosurvey in the human population. Eur J Epidemiol 1990;6:293–299.
77 Wells GM, Woodward TE, Fiset P, Hornick BB: Rocky mountain spotted fever caused by blood transfusion. J Am Med Ass 1978;239:2763–2765.
78 Arbeitskreis Blut, Untergruppe 'Bewertung Blutassoziierter Krankheitserreger': *Yersinia enterocolitica*. Bundesgesundheitsbl Gesundheitsforsch Gesundheitsschutz 1999;42:613–621.
79 Butler T, Dennis DT: Yersinia species, including plague; in Mandell GL, Bennett JE, Dolin R (eds): Principles and Practice of Infectious Diseases, 6th ed. Philadelphia, Elsevier, 2005, pp 2691–2708.
80 Prentice MB, Rahalison L: Plague. Lancet 2007;369: 1196–1207.
81 Perry RD, Fetherston JD: *Yersinia pestis* – etiologic agent of plaque. Clin Micrbiol Rev 1997;10:35–66.
82 Saikh KU, Kissner TL, Dyas B, Tropea JE, Waugh DS, Ulrich RG: Human cytolytic T cell recognition of *Yersinia pestis* virulence proteins that target innate immune response. J Infect Dis 2006;194: 1753–1760.
83 Chalton DA, Musson JA, Smith HF, Walker N, McGregor A, Lamb HK, Williamson ED, Miller J, Robinson JH, Lakey JH: Immunogenicity of a *Yersinia pestis* vaccine antigen monomerized by circular permutation. Infect Immun 2006;74: 6624–6631.
84 Chase CJ, Ulrich MP, Wasieloski LP, Kondig JP, Garrison J, Lindler LE, Kulesh DA: Real time PCR assays targeting a unique chromosomal sequence of *Yersinia pestis*. Clin Chem 2005;51:1778–1785.
85 Loiez C, Herwegh S, Wallet F, Armand S, Guinet F, Courcol RJ: Detection of *Yersinia pestis* in sputum by real-time PCR. J Clin Microbiol 2003;41: 4873–4875.

86 Tomaso H, Reisinger EC, AlDahouk S, Frangoulidis D, Rakin A, Landt O, Neubauer H: Rapid detection of *Yersinia pestis* with multiplex real-time PCR assays using fluorescent hybridisation probes. FEMS Immunol Med Microbiol 2003;38:117–126.
87 Hansmann Y, DeMartino S, Piémont Y, Meyer N, Mariet P, Heller R, Christmann D, Jaulhac B: Diagnosis of cat scratch disease with detection of *Bartonella henselae* by PCR: a study of patients with lymph node enlargement. J Clin Microbiol 2005; 43:3800–3806.
88 Simon MM, Birkner N, Lamers R, Wallich R: Outer surface lipoproteins of *Borrelia burgdorferi*: role in virulence, persistence of the pathogen and protection against Lyme disease; in Cabello FC, Hulinska D, Godfrey HP (eds): Molecular Biology of Spirochetes. Nato Science Series, I: Life and Behavioural Sciences. Fairfax, IOS Press, 2006, vol 373, pp 383–392.
89 Hepbrun MJ, Purcell BK, Lawler JV, Coyne SR, Petitt PL, Sellers KD, Norwood DA, Ulrich MP: Live vaccine strain *Francisella tularensis* is detectable at the inoculation site but not in blood after vaccination against tularaemia. Clin Infect Dis 2006;43: 711–716.
90 Pechous R, Celli J, Penoske R, Hayes SF, Frank DW, Zahrt TC: Construction and characterization of an attenuated prurine auxotroph in a *Francisella tularensis* live vaccine strain. Infect Immun 2006; 74:4452–4461.
91 Arbeitskreis Blut, Untergruppe 'Bewertung Blutassoziierter Krankheitserreger': Arboviruses – Viruses transmissible by arthropods. Transfus Med Hemother 2005;32:24–32.
92 Paddock CD, Childs JE: *Ehrlichia chaffeensis*: a prototypical emerging pathogen. Clin Microbiol Rev. 2003;16:37–64.

Impressum

Die Zeitschrift erscheint zweimonatlich; pro Jahr erscheint 1 Band zu je 6 Heften. DGTI-Mitglieder erhalten die Zeitschrift im Rahmen ihrer Mitgliedschaft. Der Bezug ist im Rahmen des Mitgliedsbeitrags abgegolten. Für den Jahrgang 36, 2009, gelten folgende Bezugspreise: Print-Abonnement EUR 169,–, Online-Abonnement EUR 169,–, Kombi-Abonnement Print/Online EUR 215,–, einschließlich MWSt., zuzüglich Postgebühren. Der Abonnementpreis ist im voraus zahlbar. Das Abonnement der Zeitschrift läuft weiter, wenn es nicht spätestens 4 Wochen vor Abschluss eines Bandes abbestellt wird. Abonnementbestellungen können bei jeder Buchhandlung oder direkt beim Verlag aufgegeben werden:

Deutschland:
S. Karger Verlag für Medizin und Naturwissenschaften GmbH
Lörracher Str. 16a
D-79115 Freiburg
Tel. +49 761 45 20 70
Fax +49 761 4 52 07 14
E-mail Information@Karger.de

Übrige Länder:
S. Karger AG
Allschwilerstr. 10
Postfach
CH-4009 Basel
Tel. +41 61 3 06 11 11
Fax +41 61 3 06 12 34
E-mail Karger@Karger.ch

Anzeigen:
S. Karger Verlag für Medizin und Naturwissenschaften GmbH
Lörracher Str. 16a
D-79115 Freiburg,
Tel. +49 761 45 20 70
Gültig ist die Preisliste Nr. 23 vom 1. Januar 2009.

Verlagsleitung und presserechtlich verantwortlich: Sibylle Hopf
Produktionsleitung: Georg Brunner
Anzeigenleitung: Susanne Meister

Gesamtherstellung:
VVA/Konkordia GmbH, 76534 Baden-Baden
Das Medienunternehmen

Bibliographische Dienste
Biological Abstracts
Current Contents/Clinical Medicine
Excerpta Medica/EMBASE
Medical Documentation Service
Reference Update
Research Alert
Science Citation Index
SCISEARCH Database

KARGER
Fax +49 761 4 52 07 14
Information@Karger.de
www.karger.com

© 2009 S. Karger GmbH, Freiburg

Accessible online at:
www.karger.com/tmh

Transfusion Medicine and Hemotherapy

Transfus Med Hemother 2009;36:79–93
DOI: 10.1159/000188082

Report of the Working Group 'Overall Blood Supply Strategy with Regard to Variant Creutzfeldt-Jakob Disease (vCJD)'

Statement on the Development and Implementation of Test Systems Suitable for the Screening of Blood Donors for vCJD – Dated September 17, 2008

Working Group 'Overall Blood Supply Strategy with Regard to Variant Creutzfeldt-Jakob Disease (vCJD)'

1 Introduction

The Working Group 'Overall Blood Supply Strategy with Regard to Variant Creutzfeldt-Jakob Disease (vCJD)' was formed in 2001 by request of the German Federal Ministry of Health in a letter dated January 26, 2001, consisting of staffs from the Paul-Ehrlich-Institut, the Robert Koch-Institut and the Federal Ministry of Health as well as external experts. On August 17, 2001 the report prepared by this Working Group was submitted to the Ministry of Health and published after a discussion in the National Advisory Committee 'Blood' (Arbeitskreis Blut) as a brochure and online [1]. After reports were published in the UK in 2004 on the transmission of the vCJD pathogen by blood transfusion, the Working Group became active again, preparing an update of the report on April 13, 2004 which was published in scientific journals [2, 3]. One of the conclusions of this report was: 'The secondary route of infection by blood could largely be stopped as soon as a suitable screening test becomes available. No such test is currently available nor is its availability foreseeable. Providing resources for developing suitable test methods should therefore be treated with high priority.' Early in 2008 the Working Group has started meeting again with slightly different members in order to assess progress made in the field of diagnostics, particularly with regard to the development of screening assays for blood donations. Another task has been to critically evaluate the requirements regarding an implementation of such test assays in the present basic framework.
The previous report of the Working Group has only been published a short time ago [2], therefore the present statement will not provide an extensive exploration of the whole set of vCJD problems again. Here we rather specifically discuss significant new aspects in the context of developing diagnostic assays. In order to illustrate the scope of the clinical difficulties, we give a brief survey on the epidemiology of vCJD and a presentation of how to clinically and diagnostically differentiate recently published borderline cases. Because the most recent development of assays has predominantly targeted the detection of pathological prion protein (PrP), new aspects of the pathophysiological impact of prions and their detectability are discussed.
Tests currently under development as well as recently published methods are presented in brief, without aiming for completeness in this treatise or for an elaborate in-depth assessment. The essential focus is rather on presenting and debating the general framework regarding the implementation of such assays. Relevant are the currently prevailing premises and the present regulation on the approval of the market access of screening tests for vCJD in Europe. Before the introduction of their widespread application in the screening of blood donors, the performance of the test assays must be thoroughly evaluated regarding their sensitivity and particularly their specificity. Preconditions of such evaluation studies in the context of implementing European regulations into the German legal system are discussed in detail. Ethical issues are particularly challenging, especially informing test persons / blood donors about a vCJD diagnosis that is still fatal, while a reliable confirmation test is lacking. At last, practical and technical requirements will be presented that must be considered on implementation.
Without putting the general aim of effectively screening of blood donors for vCJD into question, the present report of the Working Group points out considerable difficulties when implementing such assays under the prevailing preconditions. It should provide impetuses for the advancement of the handling of the assays by the regulatory bodies and for decision-making regarding the pressing ethical issues. These considerations might also be valuable for other diseases that will come into the focus in the future.

KARGER

Fax +49 761 4 52 07 14
Information@Karger.de
www.karger.com

Accessible online at:
www.karger.com/tmh

Prof. Dr. med. Rainer Seitz
Paul-Ehrlich-Institut
Paul-Ehrlich-Straße 51–59, 63225 Langen, Germany
Tel. +49 6103 77-2601, Fax -1250
E-mail seira@pei.de

Table 1. Typical characteristics of vCJD compared to sporadic CJD

	vCJD	sporadic CJD
Mean age at death	30 years	65 years
Mean duration of the disease	14 months	6 months
Clinical symptoms at the onset of disease	dysesthesia, behavioral changes	memory disorder, ataxia
EEG	non-typical	66% PSWCs
Detection of 14-3-3 protein in cerebrospinal fluid	50%	94%
Magnetic resonance tomography	hyperintensities in the thalamus, 'pulvinar sign'	hyperintensities in the basal ganglia
Codon 129 genotype	MM	MM, MV, VV
Lymphatic system	PrP^{TSE}	no PrP^{TSE}
Neuropathologic characteristics	'florid plaques'	variable, no 'florid plaques'

PSWCs = Periodic sharp and slow wave complexes.

2 Present Epidemiological Data on vCJD, Clinical and Diagnostic Differentiation from Sporadic CJD

In the early 1920s human spongiform encephalopathies were described by H.G. Creutzfeldt [4] and A. Jakob [5]. In the 1930s it could be demonstrated that scrapie, a spongiform encephalopathy of sheep and goats, is a transmissible neurodegenerative disease. Histological investigations of the brain of animals and humans who had contracted transmissible spongiform encephalopathy (TSE), using routine staining methods like hematoxylin/eosin staining, showed spongious alterations, loss of nerve cells, and in some cases amyloid accumulations. The degree of the morphological changes can vary in different regions of the brain. Therefore the diagnostic standard procedure includes the identification of the pathogen PrP^{TSE} in the brain.

2.1 Epidemiology of vCJD

This form of the disease is associated etiologically and pathogenetically with bovine spongiform encephalopathy (BSE). So far, more than 200 cases of vCJD have been reported worldwide. These patients are considerably younger than those affected by the sporadic form of CJD, and the course of the disease is prolonged (table 1). Psychiatric abnormalities are predominant (mostly in the shape of depression or psychosis) that can last for several months without any neurological signs. Later there are painful dysesthesia and walking ataxia while dementia appears only late in the course of the disease. In vCJD, the abnormal PrP can usually be also detected in the peripheral lymphatic tissues (appendix, tonsils, lymph nodes) (table 1). However, the abnormal PrP has also been found in the spleen and in muscle tissue in the sporadic form of CJD [6]. Transmissions of vCJD by blood transfusions were observed in the UK (detailed discussion in [2]). It can be considered as favorable that so far there have been no signs of an adaption of the pathogen after transmission via blood [7]. Table 2 gives a survey of the vCJD cases reported to date.

Table 2. Presently known vCJD cases, as of August 19, 2008 [8]

Country	Total number of cases	Secondary transmission (blood)	No residence in UK > 6 months
UK	166	3 (+ 1*)	
France	23		22
Republic of Ireland	4		2
Italy	1		1
USA	3		1
Canada	1		
Saudi Arabia	1		1
Japan	1		1
The Netherlands	2		2
Portugal	2		2
Spain	4		4
Total	208	3 (+ 1 *)	36

*1 case of a probable transmission of vCJD, recipient has died from other causes.

Based on a model calculation [9], in the previous report [2] the Working Group has come to the conclusion that in Germany, even in worst-case scenarios, blood transfusions would not significantly promote the possible incidence of vCJD. Therefore, the report argued against an exclusion of transfusion recipients from donating blood. Mathematic modeling studies for the UK region [10] also assume that a perpetuation of vCJD is conceivable, but improbable. According to actual calculations, the group at Imperial College in London does not consider blood transfusions to have any significant influence on the epidemiology of vCJD [11].

2.2 Clinical and Pathological Classification, Phenotype Diversity of CJD

It is crucial to be able to differentiate vCJD which has evidentially been transmitted by blood from other forms of human

Table 3. Phenotypical CJD characteristics

	Molecular subtype	Clinical features	Neuropathology	PrP immunohistochemistry
Frequent	MM1/MV1	dementia, cortical anopsy, myoclonia, short duration of disease (approximately 4 months)	pronounced damage of the occipital cortex, PrP accumulations of the synaptic type	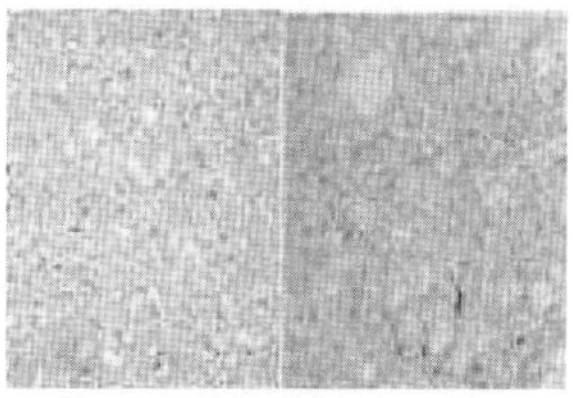
	MV2	ataxia, dementia, extrapyramidal motion disorder, long duration of disease (approximately 18 months)	focal damage of the cortex, amyloid (kuru) plaques, focal plaque-like PrP accumulations	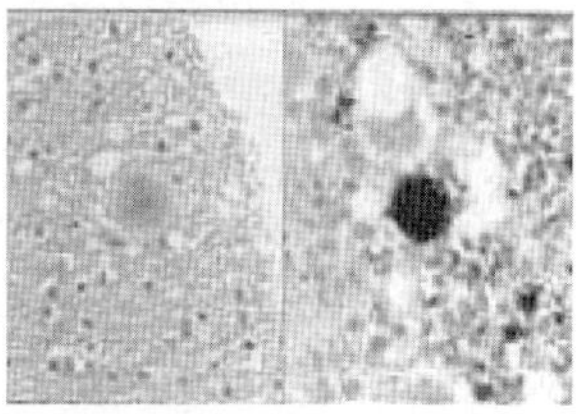
	VV2	ataxia at onset, dementia at a late stage, average duration of disease (approximately 7 months)	pronounced damage of the subcortical structures as well as the brainstem, often spongiosis only located in the deeper cortical layers, plaque-like as well as perineuronal PrP accumulations	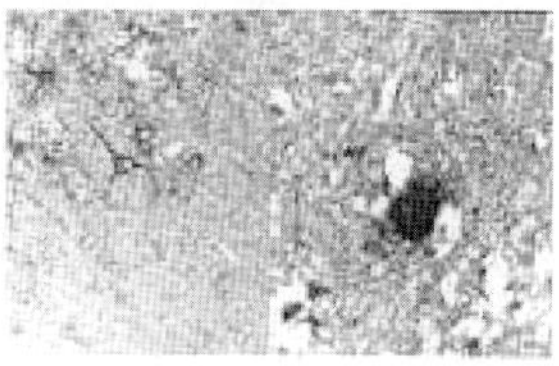
Rare	MM2 thalamic (sFI)	insomnia, dysautonomia, at a late stage ataxia and cognitive disturbance	atrophy of the thalamus and the nucleus olivaris, lack of spongiosis possible	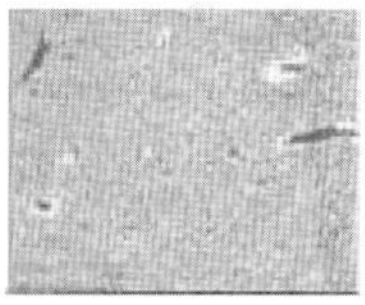
	MM2 cortical	dementia for several months	large confluent vacuoles with perivacuolar PrP accumulations	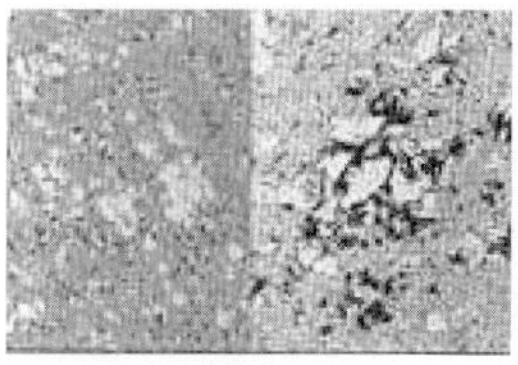
	VV1	dementia at onset, later ataxia and extrapyramidal disorders	spongiosis, gliosis and loss of innervation of the cortical structures while omitting the brainstem and the cerebellum	
vCJD	MM2b	psychiatric, dysaesthesia, ataxia, later dementia	spongiosis, gliosis and loss of innervation as well as 'florid' plaques	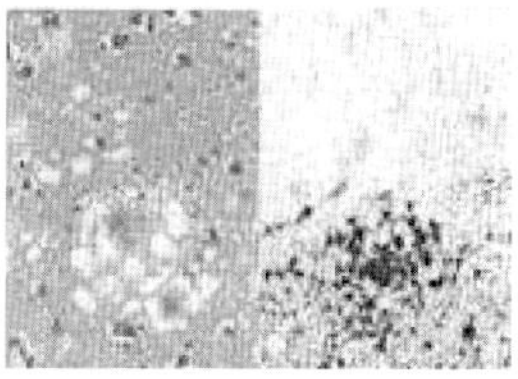

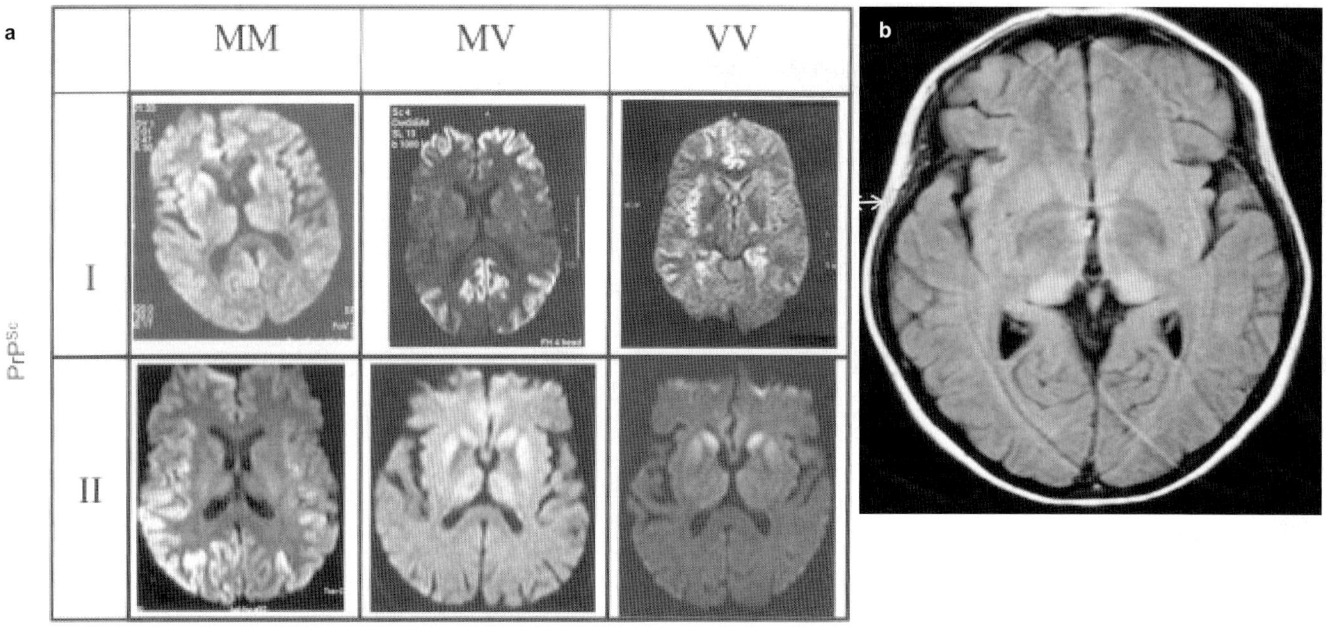

Fig. 1. a Patterns of lesions by MRT in sporadic CJD – differences in the molecular subtypes (weighting of diffusion). **b** Alterations in MRT in vCJD – increased signal in the posterior thalamus (FLAIR [fluid attenuated inversion recovery] imaging). The image has kindly been provided by Dr D. Collie, Western General Hospital, Edinburgh, UK.

TSE for which there are as yet no indications for a transmissibility by blood. To illustrate this difficulty induced by the diversity in phenotype, some cases will be discussed here in detail. Recently, Mead et al. [12] have reported a CJD in a 39-year-old female patient who first consulted a physician in January of 1999 because of visual disturbance. She then developed cognitive impairment, halting gait, motility disorder of the eye, dysarthria, stereotypical movements and myoclonia as well as finally progressive ataxia and dementia. 14 months after the onset of the disease the patient died. The codon 129 genotype was homozygous for valine. In this subtype (most often molecular VV2 subtype) ataxia is prominent while there are also signs of cognitive impairment, tonus abnormalities, and myoclonia. Typical characteristics are the lack of periodic sharp and slow wave complexes, as also happened in this patient, as well as the detection of the 14-3-3 proteins in the cerebrospinal fluid. Magnetic resonance tomography (MRT) is compatible with this subtype in which often a symmetrical affection of the basal ganglia without cortical involvement is found (unpublished data). A report in the journal *New Scientist* [13] cites the first author, Simon Mead, as follows: 'The consensus is that it's more likely sporadic, but we can't conclude either way until further experiments are done.' The overall course of disease is compatible with sporadic CJD, as observed in molecular VV2 subtype (compare table 3), regarding the development of clinical symptoms, the results of additional technical investigations, and the duration of the disease.

Gambetti et al. [14] have recently described a novel degenerative brain disease in humans that is associated with abnormal PrP. The disease occurred in patients of a mean age of 62 years and is clinically characterized by rapidly progredient cognitive disturbances as well as movement disorder. The clinical phase has a mean duration of 20 months. Brain tissue obtained by autopsy (10 patients) or by biopsy (1 patient) was investigated histologically and showed spongiform degeneration, astrogliosis and in some of the cases 'micro-plaque'-like accumulations of the PrP and, after immunohistochemical staining, pronounced granular accumulations of the PrP. On the biochemical level there was comparatively little abnormal PrP that was less highly aggregated and the proteinase K(PK)-sensitive fraction of which was considerably larger than that in sporadic CJD. In addition, during enzymatic proteolysis the protein forms different protease-resistant cleavage products than those in the case of the well-known forms of CJD.

One year earlier a new subtype of CJD had been reported in Germany [15] that showed similarities to the above-mentioned cases described by Gambetti et al. [14]. The reports prompted a search for similar patients within the cohort of the German national reference center. So far, this search was unsuccessful.

Regardless of the above-described cases that are difficult to classify, the molecular classification of sporadic CJD is based on the codon 129 genotype of the PrP gene (homozygous for methionine (MM) or valine (VV), or heterozygous (MV)) and on the biochemical properties of the abnormal PrP (PrP^{TSE} type 1 or 2, differentiated by size and migration rate of the unglycosylized PrP band in the immunoblot). The molecular subtypes of the disease are accompanied by distinct clinical and neuropathological phenotypes of CJD (table 3).

MRT proves to be a diagnostic technique by which it is possible to differentiate individual CJD subtypes from each other and

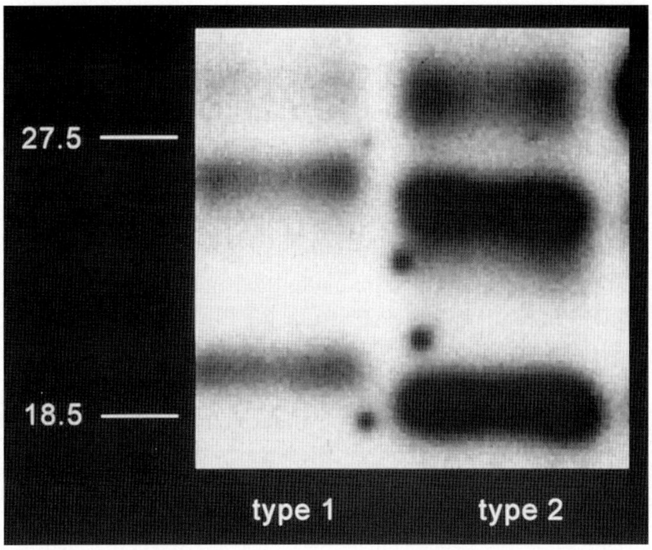

Fig. 2. PrP^{TSE} types 1 and 2 in isoforms of sporadic CJD in Western Blot.

from vCJD, even before death. In addition, it is instrumental in identifying atypical courses of the disease at a very early stage (fig. 1a, b).

2.3 *Typing of PrP^{TSE}*

Cerebellar tissue of the patient that was homozygous for valine at codon 129 of the *PRNP* gene [12] was investigated by Western Blot in order to type PrP^{TSE}. Differences to well-known PrP^{TSE} types of sporadic CJD isoforms (fig. 2) became apparent. The relative proportion and electrophoretic migration pattern of the di-, mono- and unglycosylated bands of the PK-digested PrP^{TSE} were more similar to the PrP^{TSE} type found in vCJD. In contrast to vCJD-associated PrP^{TSE}, the addition of EDTA (a chelating agent binding copper and zinc ions) to the PK digestion of the patient's PrP^{TSE} caused a further slight reduction in the molecular weight of the three protein bands. From the results of their Western Blot investigations the authors concluded that the pathological PrP of the patient investigated represents a novel PrP^{TSE} type that is different from PrP^{TSE} types so far observed in sporadic CJD cases. Furthermore the three-dimensional structure differs from that displayed in vCJD-associated PrP^{TSE} (from patients with MM at the *PRNP* codon 129). The authors classify the newly described PrP^{TSE} type as 'type 7' in their classification system which is being developed over the past years. However, most experts prefer PrP^{TSE} typing according to Parchi et al. [16]. According to this system, there are two basic PrP^{TSE} types associated with sporadic CJD and one PrP^{TSE} type associated with vCJD. Parchi et al. [16] were able to show that even minimal variations of the experimental conditions (e.g. the pH value) in PK digestion have considerable impact on the size of the resulting PrP^{TSE} fragments and may possibly generate artificial PrP^{TSE} types. In order to be able to assess the results by Mead et al. [12], it would therefore be helpful if the investigations could be reproduced using the method by Parchi et al. [16] under exactly defined pH and buffer conditions. On the one hand, by such investigations the slight difference in molecular weight could be additionally corroborated which is observed after EDTA treatment compared to the vCJD-associated PrP^{TSE} type. On the other hand, this might also lead to a better understanding of the results shown in figure 4c in [12]. In this figure the PrP^{TSE} of the patient after EDTA treatment and PK conspicuously resembles PrP^{TSE} type 3 rather than the new type 7 – unlike the one shown in lane 2 of figure 4b in [12].

It is not possible to deduce from the published Western Blot data of a single case whether the newly described PrP^{TSE} type is in any way connected with the BSE agent. Only transmission experiments in transgenic or normal mice might shed more light on a more precise characterization of the agent strain, allowing a continued sensitive epidemiological surveillance of the CJD trends.

3 New Aspects of the Pathophysiology and the Diagnostics of Prions

In 1985 the PrP was identified as a gene product [17]. Since it is also found in healthy organisms, it is essential to be able to differentiate between the normal or cellular PrP, called PrP^{C}, and the pathogenic infectious isoform, called PrP^{TSE} in this report. Both forms of PrP, PrP^{C} and PrP^{TSE}, display the same composition of amino acids [18] and glycosylation pattern as well as the same lipid anchor because both proteins are coded by the same gene. The differences between PrP^{C} and PrP^{TSE} lie in their structural and physicochemical properties that are assumed to be responsible for infectivity. These properties permit the development of diagnostic assays for PrP^{TSE}:

- Isolated PrP^{C} is water soluble, whereas PrP^{TSE} cannot be dissolved (without losing its infectivity).
- PrP^{C} predominantly contains α-helices as its secondary structural element, whereas PrP^{TSE} displays a high proportion of β-sheet structures [19, 20]. Conversion of PrP^{C} to PrP^{TSE} renders the PrP infectious.
- PK treatment rapidly digests PrP^{C} to oligopeptides, whereas in the case of PrP^{TSE} PK treatment leads to the cleaving off of an N-terminal part of the PrP that is 68 amino acids in length. The cleavage site differs among the various prion strains and is located approximately between amino acid positions 87 and 107. The remaining molecule has a (strain-specific) molecular weight of around 27–30 kDa which is the reason why it is also called PrP27-30. For hours it resists further PK digestion which is true for almost every prion strain. Therefore, the presence or absence of pathological PK-resistant PrP^{TSE} in tissue homogenates can be detected by Western Blot, for example. The PK concentration in these experiments must be high enough for a complete digestion of PrP^{C}.

- High molecular PrP^{TSE} aggregates can also be detected in infected tissues, e.g. as amyloid plaques. In tissue homogenates aggregates can be separated from cellular, nonaggregated PrP^{C}, i.e. by centrifugation, and be enriched in the sediment. Treatment with e.g. phosphotungstic acid can increase sedimentation [21].

Using immunohistochemistry, the misfolded PrP^{TSE} is detected not only in a variety of plaques (kuru plaque, multicentric and florid plaques) but also in additional structures. The precondition for an immunohistochemical detection of PrP^{TSE} is a denaturing pretreatment of the tissue sections samples (e.g. formic acid or guanidinium thiocyanate treatment) so that cellular PrP^{C} can no longer be displayed. Additional treatment of the histological sections with PK can lead to an even more pronounced visibility of PrP^{TSE}. The immunohistochemical methods are based on antibodies against the PrP, either in the form of polyclonal sera or of monoclonal antibodies (MABs); the latter are almost exclusively used today. As mentioned above, the composition of amino acids and the glycosylation pattern of PrP^{C} and PrP^{TSE} are identical, therefore no immunological or inflammatory reactions can be detected, either during the incubation stage or after clinical symptoms have developed. This explains the lack of serological detection methods like for other pathogens. Preferably knock-out mice that do not express PrP, so-called $PrP^{0/0}$ mice, are used for the development of MABs. The best-known MABs are 3F4 [22] (reaction with human and hamster PrP), 13A5 [23] (reaction with hamster PrP) and 6H4 [24] (reaction with human, bovine, ovine, mouse and hamster PrP). These MABs bind to both PrP^{C} and (denatured) PrP^{TSE} so that a differentiation between cellular and pathogenic isoforms of the PrP becomes possible only after using additional diagnostic methods, e.g. PK digestion of PrP^{C} as used for the Western Blot. So far, only few MABs have been described that selectively recognize PrP^{TSE} due to the reaction with a conformational epitope. One of these is MAB 15B3 [24], a MAB of the IgM class. Above all, this MAB is used for precipitation and concentration of PrP^{TSE}, while no additional properties of this MAB have yet been described. In the meantime, further conformation-specific MABs have been described [25–27]. Several MABs that were described to be PrP^{TSE}-specific apparently react with aggregated infectious and noninfectious PrP [28]. Binding of PrP^{TSE} can be achieved by means of MABs coupled to 'microbeads'; apparently MAB specificity does not play a role here [29].

In addition to detecting PrPs by antibody-binding reactions, the (differences in the) glycosylation pattern can be used for discriminating prion strains according to their lectin-binding properties [30]. A PK treatment is required for such a differentiation because the binding to lectin in sporadic CJD is mainly detectable in the non-cleaved PrP while in vCJD the PK-treated PrP also shows a strong reaction.

The correlation of infectivity with an immunohistochemical detection of PrP^{TSE} in animal experiments (generally using intracerebral application of brain homogenate or homogenates of other tissues such as spleen) has led to the conclusion that immunohistochemical proof of PrP^{TSE} in fact confirms a TSE disease. Differentiation of the cellular (nonpathogenic) isoform PrP^{C} from the (pathogenic) isoform PrP^{TSE} is crucial since currently this represents the only diagnostic marker. It must be kept in mind that, in the case of a TSE disease, PrP^{TSE} must be specifically identified in a background of PrP^{C} present in a concentration that is several magnitudes higher. Several methods that are described below are under development which should allow differentiating of PrP^{C} from PrP^{TSE} for diagnostic purposes.

So far, the established methods for diagnosing a TSE disease like CJD or vCJD are based on either immunohistopathological investigations or Western Blotting. In order to be able to identify PrP^{TSE} by these methods, denaturing and/or proteolytic cleavage of PrP^{C} are required. The presently widely used conformation-dependent immunoassay (CDI) [21] represents the only method to specifically identify PrP^{TSE} even in a background of high concentrations of PrP^{C}. With this method even PK-sensitive PrP^{TSE} could be detected in the brain of patients with sporadic CJD [31]. However, these methods are restricted to post-mortem diagnostics or to tissue biopsies.

Resistance of pathogenic PrP^{TSE} against PK digestion has long been known not to be absolute but rather dependent on the prion strain, too. For example, strain DROWSY (DY) is sensitive to PK digestion, in contrast to other strains including strain HYPER (HY) [32]. DY and HY are prion strains that cause transmissible encephalopathy of the mink (TME) and that have been further passaged in hamsters. As has been observed in strain DY, infectivity of PrP^{TSE} is not associated with PK resistance of the PrP. Therefore some authors also use the terms $sPrP^{TSE}$ (PK-sensitive PrP^{TSE}) and $rPrP^{TSE}$ (PK-resistant PrP^{TSE}). Investigations of brain samples from patients with CJD have shown that more than 80% of total PrP^{TSE} is PK-resistant [31]. Additional investigations in mice have confirmed an infectivity that is associated with PK-sensitive PrP^{TSE} [33]. These investigations have used prion strains in which only small amounts of PrP^{TSE} could be demonstrated by immunohistochemistry. Here a high infectivity titer was found (more than 10^7 infectious units/g of brain homogenate), but no PK-resistant PrP^{TSE}. However, it must be taken into consideration that the sensitivity of the Western Blot was comparatively low: the detection limit was 25 µg PrP^{TSE}/g of wet weight.

In case PrP^{TSE} isolated from brain homogenate is purified by differential centrifugation, and the supernatant is investigated for infectivity after high-speed centrifugation (220,000 × g for 30 min), only a minimal amount (if any) of PrP^{TSE} can be demonstrated by Western Blot, but high infectivity titers. In this case also, infectivity seems to be associated mainly with PK-sensitive PrP^{TSE} (an at least 200- to 1,000-fold higher infectivity titer than expected from the biochemical signal (Western Blot) has been described [34]). It is noteworthy that the low PrP^{TSE} signal in Western Blot could be precipitated quantitatively with phosphotungstic acid, together with the whole amount of infectivity of the sample. This precipitation step can also be usefully applied in precipitating PK-resistant PrP^{TSE} [21, 35]. It remains to be clarified to what extent this PrP preparation, present in the high-speed centrifugation supernatant, consists (only) of low molecular PrP^{TSE} aggregates showing a very high specific infectivity. For example, it was reported that oligomers consisting of 14–28 PrP^{TSE} molecules exhibit the highest infectivity. The molecular weight of these oligomers ranges between 300 and 600 kDa, and their size is between 17 and 27 nm. Oligomers consisting of as little as 5 PrP^{TSE} molecules or less do not seem to be infectious [36].

Endogenous infectivity in the blood of experimentally infected animals can be demonstrated not only in the clinical but already in the preclinical stage of a TSE disease [37–41]. At least part of this infectivity is PK-sensitive [42]. An incubation of the endogenous infectivity in plasma with different concentrations of PK (100 and 500 µg) reduces the infectivity titer from 20.6 in the control without PK down to 8.4 and 5.2 infectious units/ml, respectively. However, it must be stated that the PK concentrations investigated were insufficient for a complete digestion of plasma proteins. Therefore, it cannot be excluded that a PK concentration sufficiently high for a complete proteolysis of plasma proteins would also have completely digested the infectivity in the plasma samples.

As mentioned above, to some extent infectivity can be PK-sensitive. Therefore, it must be pointed out that diagnostic assays using PK digestion for differentiation might miss part of the infectious PrP^{TSE} and might thus prevent correct diagnostic conclusions.

4 Development of Diagnostic Assays

In statements regarding measures to prevent the transmission of vCJD via blood and blood products, various countries have addressed the necessity of developing diagnostic assays for the identification of vCJD infectivity in the blood. For example, the Working Group 'Overall Blood Supply Strategy with Regard to Variant Creutzfeldt-Jakob Disease (vCJD)' in their statement dated April 13, 2006 [2] pointed out that the development of screening assays was one of the key issues in preventing possible transmissions of vCJD by blood products, and in initiating therapeutic measures – supposed they would be available – at an early stage of infection. If a direct identification of vCJD-infected blood donors by screening assays was to become possible already in the incubation period, testing of donations would be particularly superior to any indirect measures that lack specificity, such as the prophylactic exclusion of groups of donors with an elevated risk in their history.

The major difficulty in developing such assays is the very low concentration of PrP^{TSE} that is to be expected, in a background of the physiological PrP^{C} that is present at an approximately 10,000-fold surplus. The analytical sensitivity of screening assays that seem to be appropriate for the detection of PrP^{TSE} in serum or plasma must be far lower than 1 pg/ml PrP^{TSE} [2]. Assuming that in an infected brain one infectious unit corresponds to approximately 0.01–1.0 µg, the required sensitivity of the assay would have to correspond to approximately 1–100 nl of a 10% brain homogenate [43]. Additional requirements are high specificity, robustness as well as applicability in blood donation testing.

The UK National Institute for Biological Standards and Control (NIBSC) provides a plasma panel containing variable amounts of infectious and noninfectious material from the brain or spleen of patients with vCJD (NIBSC CJD Research Centre, Plasma Panel, Reference code NHPM0/0015: Normal Human Plasma spiked with vCJD Ctrl Brain/Spleen, 22 tubes, concentration range). This as well as other panels have already been used in a comparative assessment of tests under development. In 2007 Phil Minor has reported the results of an external quality assessment involving seven laboratories using eight test assays. Four out of eight assays were able to detect ≤100 nl of a 10% brain homogenate containing the vCJD agent while three other assays detected <300 nl [43]. At a hearing of the DG Enterprise (Directorate General Enterprise and Industry) on October 27, 2007 in Brussels a company announced that they were aiming to obtain the CE marking for a test assay still in 2008 [44].

In the context of an epidemiological investigation, the British health authorities stated on February 6, 2007 their intention to test 60,000 plasma samples [45]. Companies were requested to provide assays for these investigations. As a first step in selecting an assay for these investigations, the comparative assessment of a plasma panel was performed by an independent laboratory. While the comparative assessment has been finished, the epidemiological investigation has not yet started.

Because the development of diagnostic assays is progressing considerably, it has become necessary to clearly determine which specific requirements should be made on a test able to detect vCJD in blood and which materials could be provided to characterize such an assay.

Currently various diagnostic assays are being developed, using different approaches. Such methods are based e.g. on binding to specific ligands, on the application of antibodies, on the detection or induction of conformation changes as well as on PCR-like protein amplification. Some of these assays will be briefly presented in the following.

4.1 Conformation-Dependent Immunoassay (CDI)

Detection of PrP^{TSE} by CDI (originating from S. Prusiner's laboratory) uses the approach of 'epitope exposure' [21, 31]: defined epitopes that are at first inaccessible in the native PrP^{TSE} are exposed by denaturation, followed by detection using a Europium-labeled antibody. Last year, at the conference 'Prion 2007' in Edinburgh, J. Safar reported that this assay was able to detect PrP^{TSE} in LDL (low density lipoprotein) fractions in plasma from patients with sporadic CJD. For 20 patients with sCJD a sensitivity of the assay of 90% was found, while specificity was 98 and 95% using control samples from 103 normal blood donors and from 20 donors with dementia of other etiology (like e.g. Alzheimer's disease), respectively.

4.2 *Misfolded Protein Diagnostic (MPD) Assay*

To specifically detect PrP^{TSE}, this assay employs a pyrene-labeled palindromic sequence of prion peptides. As their characteristic molecular structural element, pyrene and its derivatives possess a conjugated aromatic system of four fused benzene rings. They are used among other things as dyes and as molecular probes in fluorescence spectroscopy. A palindrome is a row of signs that, on reading forward as well as backward, result in the same sequence of signs. The peptide employed in the MPD assay undergoes a cascade of coil to β-sheet conversion in the presence of PrP^{TSE}, accompanied by a measurable fluorescence shift of the dye. In a blinded study using the MPD assay it was possible to detect PrP^{TSE} in the plasma of 5 patients with sporadic CJD while the assay gave negative results for the plasma from 5 normal donors [46].

4.3 *Epitope Protection Assay*

This assay is based on the modification of amino acids of the PrP by reaction with free radicals that are released by chemical reactions. This results in the destruction of specific epitopes on the surface that can no longer be recognized by antibodies. Because the pathogenic PrP^{TSE} is present in an aggregated form, part of the protein is protected against reaction with free radicals. Epitopes are thus preserved that can then react with monoclonal antibodies which allows to detect PrP^{TSE} after disintegration of the aggregates in the immunoassay. The assay employs magnetic beads loaded with antibodies and is supposed to be able to detect less than 10 fg recombinant PrP^{TSE} in the sample.

4.4 *PMCA-Based Detection of PrP^{TSE}*

In 2001 Soto and colleagues [47] have published the 'Protein Misfolding Cyclic Amplification' (PMCA) as a method to amplify pathologically aggregated PrP in vitro. PrP^{TSE}, the disease-associated form of the PrP, is first incubated in a surplus of normal, nonaggregated PrP^{C}. Seeded nucleus-induced polymerization integrates PrP into available PrP^{TSE} aggregates, causing them to virtually 'grow'. Using sonication, these enlarged PrP^{TSE} aggregates are then fragmented into smaller parts which in turn can function again as 'matrices' or 'nuclei' in another PMCA cycle. It is unclear whether such reaction products are infectious; in case they are, special safety measures would be required.

Recently, Atarashi et al. [48, 49] have reported to have enhanced the PMCA technique resulting in the *QUIC Assay* which is supposed to allow a considerably more rapid and feasible detection of PrP^{TSE} than conventional PMCA methods. By employing recombinant PrP as a substrate, incubating the samples at elevated temperatures and shaking (instead of sonication), the procedure is supposed to enable the detection of approximately 1 infectious unit in 24 h. The QUIC Assay was able to discriminate between scrapie-infected and uninfected hamsters using cerebrospinal fluid. The procedure has only been described for the hamster model so far.

4.5 *Amyloid Seeding Assay (ASA)*

Colby et al. [50] have developed a method to induce polymerization of recombinant PrP into amyloid fibrils by using PrP^{TSE} aggregates as seeds. The term 'amyloid' designates protein accumulations of diverse origin that can be detected in the light microscope and that share the following characteristics: i) fibrillary ultrastructure, ii) affinity to the dye Congo red, and iii) characteristic β-sheet structures. The PrP amyloid produced in the ASA is detected by binding to the dye thioflavin T (that shows a fluorescence shift after the binding). With the aid of ASA it was possible to detect PrP^{TSE} in diluted brain homogenates from patients with sporadic CJD as well as in a variety of prion strains passaged in both mice and hamsters. Conservatively estimated, the detection limit for PrP^{TSE} in the ASA is supposed to be ≤1 fg, and test results are obtained within 24 h.

4.6 *Cell Panel Assay*

Mahal et al. [51] described a cell culture assay with four cell lines that have varying susceptibility to infections with mouse-adapted prion strains RML, 22L, Me7 (scrapie-associated agents) and 301C (BSE-associated agent). The assay allows to detect and discriminate these prion strains within 2 weeks. As yet, the application of the Cell Panel Assay is relatively limited because the susceptibility of the cell lines is confined to murine prion strains.

4.7 *Detection of Prions in Organotypic Brain Slice Cultures*

Falsig et al. [52] used the so-called 'POSCA' (prion organotypic slice culture assay) for ex vivo replication and titration of the prions that are to be detected. Organotypic slices from the cerebellum of PrP-overexpressing tga20 mice were incubated in cultures for extended periods of time. 35 days after contact with prion-containing material ($scrapie^{RML}$ brain homogenate), mouse cerebellar slices had amplified PrP^{TSE} $>10^5$-fold, as shown by Western Blot. Other prion strains (79A, 139A, Me7 (scrapie-associated agents) and 301C (BSE-associated agent)) also showed PrP^{TSE} amplification using POSCA, but with variable efficiency. However, for mouse-adapted agents of the chronic wasting disease (CWD) as well as other defined scrapie strains, tga20-POSCA gave negative results. The range of application of the assay might be considerably expanded because organotypic brain slice cultures can be established from mice with the required genotypes as well as from a variety of different host species.

4.8 Atomic Dielectric Resonance Spectroscopy (ADRS)

Fagge et al. [53] have used ADRS to determine dielectric characteristics of sample material with the help of radio/micro waves in order to analyze blood samples from CJD and vCJD patients and identify characteristic 'ADR signatures' in the blood. In a preliminary study using unblinded samples from normal blood donors and from patients with vCJD, sCJD as well as other neurological diseases, initially group-specific ADRS properties were determined, and statistic analysis systems were trained to classify unknown samples. In a subsequent study employing these analysis systems it was possible to correctly classify ten blinded samples (four of them vCJD, three sCJD, three other neurological diseases). The investigations show that on the molecular level differences between the blood samples from the different groups of donors can be identified, but these differences cannot be specified. Moreover, the authors point out that it will be necessary to further verify their results in considerably larger studies.

5 Evaluation and Market Access of vCJD Screening Assays

5.1 Regulation of in vitro Diagnostic Medical Devices in Europe

It is one of the aims of the development of specific vCJD assays to identify potential carriers of vCJD already by blood screening on the occasion of blood donation and to eliminate their donation in time. Thus these assays would be applied similar to virus screening tests already widely in use by blood donation services, e.g. anti-HIV-1/-2 screening assays.

In Europe virus diagnostics for infections with HIV, HBV, HCV and HTLV, so-called high-risk products, are regulated considerably more stringently than other diagnostics, due to the in vitro diagnostic medical devices (IVDs) directive [54]. The reasons behind this classification are the severe consequences of false test results, for those concerned as well as for third parties, for example in the case of transmission of these viruses by blood transfusion to other persons due to false-negative test results of the blood donor. Regarding those IVDs not classified as high-risk products, the manufacturers are given as much of a free hand as possible to assess the state of the art on their own responsibility and to declare by CE marking the marketability of the products within the Common Market of Europe. In the case of high-risk products a thorough examination by an independent institution (Notified Body) is foreseen. Specific quality requirements, the Common Technical Specifications (CTS), must be met. In addition, before reaching the European market, the product batches are also counterchecked in an independent laboratory (batch release testing).

Regarding the risk potential, diagnostic assays for vCJD intended to be used in the blood service will have to take a position similar to anti-HIV-1/-2 screening assays: Release or exclusion of a blood donation is directly dependent on each test result. Any false-negative test results might have severe consequences for recipients of blood transfusions. Any reactive and potentially false-positive test results would require extensive investigations to clarify these results, as far as this was possible at all for vCJD diagnostic assays. Furthermore, reactive test results would represent a heavy psychological burden for the donor. It has to be mentioned that the IVD directive has been written at a time when neither the disease vCJD was known nor diagnostic assays for vCJD-infected individuals were conceivable.

A formal application to the European Commission is required in order to include new diagnostic assays into list A (high-risk products), as has been explained in detail in article 14 of the directive 98/79/EG. After some preliminary discussions, it was left to UK – being the member state most affected by vCJD – to file an application to include vCJD diagnostic assays into list A, annex 2, of the IVD directive. Such an application was filed in 2007 and is supported by several other member states, among them Germany and France. At a public hearing in Brussels dated October 26, 2007, such a classification of vCJD assays was also supported by the European IVD manufacturing industry (European Diagnostic Manufacturers Association; EDMA) and the European Medicines Agency (EMEA). As long as list A of the IVD directive has not been expanded – the application filed for this according to article 14 [54] can still take years until an official decision is made – vCJD assays can be CE-marked without special requirements and marketed in the Common Market, even for application in blood donation screening. This widely unregulated situation is very alarming.

On the occasion of the public hearing in Brussels it became also apparent that the development of CTS regarding vCJD assays will be urgently needed. A significant step would have to be experimental assessment of the assays using well-characterized samples with known vCJD infectivity. This endeavor appears to be quite difficult because such reference samples for vCJD are not available due to the low number of cases. In the meantime efforts have been made to collect the scant sample material and to systematically make it available (see below). It will be inevitable to also include other sample material, such as samples from TSE animal models, in an initial validation of diagnostic assays for the detection of vCJD in human blood. Anyway, a simple transfer of those CTS already established for current virus screening assays to the newly developed vCJD assays is not possible for several reasons. Another problem is the required testing of clinical samples in respect of sensitivity. For example, at least 400 different positive patient samples are mandatory for a sensitivity trial of the various virus screening assays, without missing any sample. Certainly this criterion is not applicable at present to vCJD assays because such sample numbers are not available.

Investigating the specificity of such assays would also be difficult. A minimal specificity of 99.5% is required in the CTS for virus screening assays. The specificity of blood screening assays has to be determined using samples from 5,000 blood donors. By definition, an investigation has a false-positive result if an initially reactive test is repeatedly reactive using the same sample and if comparable control or confirmation tests have negative results. Also there must be no further indication of a corresponding infection (e.g. clinical symptoms) for the person concerned. To implement a novel diagnostic assay without a control or confirmation test would imply that it would be impossible to differentiate false-positive from correct true-positive test results in a population that is not well characterized. Therefore, it is almost impossible at present to estimate the specificity of a vCJD assay. CTS further require the investigation of samples from hospitalized patients and samples with potentially cross-reacting components. Regarding vCJD assays, an investigation of individuals with neurological diseases for whom vCJD has been ruled out seems to be indicated. It has to be discussed further to what extent the etiological agents of other human TSE diseases may or even should cross-react.

In the UK a committee composed of international experts has been appointed at NIBSC (vCJD Repository Oversight Committee) that develops criteria for making available to manufacturers of diagnostic assays the samples registered and stored in the 'vCJD repository' of NIBSC. The Paul-Ehrlich-Institut is part of the Oversight Committee and has decided to add samples from vCJD-infected primates that were collected in the context of an EU research project at the Paul-Ehrlich-Institut to this vCJD repository at NIBSC. Thus IVD manufacturers are offered a contact point and a procedure to obtain appropriate samples that are provided under generally accepted conditions. NIBSC has already asked one manufacturer to make their diagnostic assay available for validation investigations [55]. Future CTS for vCJD assays will certainly have to also be coordinated with this policy.

Regardless of the obvious difficulties, the attempt must be made to define mandatory quality criteria also for vCJD assays, whether in the form of CTS or otherwise.

5.2 Legal and Ethical Aspects Regarding the Development and Application of Diagnostic Assays

Performance evaluation studies involving test persons and patients are necessary for an evaluation of novel IVDs. In the case of validating vCJD screening assays this would also include the testing of blood donors. Many difficult questions arise, not only in the context of these studies but also on implementing such assays into routine screening of blood donors. The set of problems under scrutiny here is particularly complex. The particular situation in Germany including the basic legal aspects and ethical implications (sources of information regarding the regulations and legislation are listed there) is discussed in detail in 'Legal and Ethical Aspects Regarding the Development and Application of Screening Assays to Detect vCJD Infections' (see online supplemental material at www.karger.com/doi/10.1159/000188082).

In summary the following should be noted:

a) Performance evaluations of IVDs are aimed at obtaining CE certification and thus marketability of such medicinal devices in the EU. Their purpose is to determine the safety and qualification of the IVDs for the intended application.
b) In order to ensure health protection for the population, in accordance with section 5 paragraph 1 Transfusion Act (Transfusionsgesetz; TFG), IVDs that allow the detection of grave and epidemiologically significant infectious diseases have to be employed to determine the eligibility of a person to donate blood. This applies under the precondition that IVDs are technically safe and suitable and that sufficient safety cannot be reached by other measures (e.g. donor exclusion). However, in view of the presently known epidemiological situation of vCJD in Germany, in view of only four confirmed transmissions by blood transfusion in the UK and in view of the difficulties described above regarding performance evaluation, the implementation of vCJD diagnostic assays appears to be inadvisable at present.
c) The performance evaluation study of an IVD for the detection of vCJD infections regularly requires the informed consent of the participant, see § 24 paragraph 1 Medical Devices Act (Medizinproduktegesetz; MPG). The only conceivable exception would be the investigation of factually anonymized samples from those individuals who are not at the same time donors in terms of the TFG, who are not suspected to carry any other disease and whose blood samples were taken for other reasons than performance evaluation studies.
d) Already in the case of a 'justifiable suspicion' of a donor to be infected with vCJD, the physician responsible is obligated to eliminate the donation, to trace and inform as well as examine any recipients and to inform the authorities responsible, unless there is a reasonable assumption of its probably being a false-positive result (see also section 19 paragraph 1 sentence 1 and sentences 6–8 as well as section 3 TFG). In view of the largely unknown epidemiology of the vCJD infection, the latter assumption cannot be justified by statistical considerations alone. Rather it has to use as definitive guidance the sensitivity and specificity (to be supported by performance evaluation studies) as well as technical feasibility of the assays to be developed for detecting a vCJD infection. On the condition that there was

a vCJD assay available, the fact alone that as yet there was no assay for confirmation or exclusion of a reactive vCJD screening test result, would be no sufficient reason to exclude a 'justifiable suspicion' for a vCJD infection in terms of the TFG, section19 paragraph 1 sentence 1.

e) In investigations carried out in the context of or on the occasion of blood donation, employing an IVD to detect a vCJD infection, a positive result implies the duty of the physician responsible to inform and counsel the donor on this fact, provided that it must be assumed that the IVD has to be regarded as able to 'confirm' a vCJD infection (see also TFG, section 19 paragraph 1 sentence 4). In this regard it firstly depends on the respective state of development of the IVD whether it can be regarded as suitable for allowing a confirmed diagnosis of a vCJD infection, even at this early stage during performance evaluation studies. According to the current state of scientific knowledge, this cannot yet be answered affirmatively in view of the vCJD diagnostic assays under development.

f) In case a positive test result is disclosed, the person concerned must receive counseling and advice by a physician, see also TFG, section 19 paragraph 1 sentence 5. But it must be taken into account that currently no diagnostic method is established to confirm a positive screening test result ante mortem and no therapy to treat or cure the terminal vCJD disease.

g) On request, participants in a performance evaluation study regarding an IVD for detecting vCJD must be informed about the test results, see sections 19 and 34 Federal Data Protection Law (Bundesdatenschutzgesetz; BDSG). In this connection they must be informed before and after participation that a positive test result does not mean in every case that they are infected with vCJD and, even if they should actually be infected, that no statement can be made regarding the question of whether the disease will become symptomatic. Furthermore they should be offered counsel and help.

h) The application of screening assays for detecting vCJD infections may have a negative effect on the general willingness to donate blood, but this fact is no adequate reason to interfere with performance evaluation studies or with the implementation of an IVD to detect vCJD infections in blood donations, at any rate unless such an infection of blood donors and in blood products can be excluded by other diagnostic methods.

i) Before performance evaluation studies of an IVD can be started, ethics boards must be involved either because of section 24 paragraph 1 in conjunction with section 20 paragraphs 7 and 8 of the MPG and/or because of legal guidelines for physicians (see section 15 of the Medical Association's professional code of conduct).

6 General Conditions and Problems Expected to Arise on Implementation of vCJD Screening Assays

6.1 Sensitivity

Due to the scarcity of human samples, the stage of development of the diagnostic assays so far does not allow any statement on their sensitivity regarding detection of vCJD in the preclinical stage. A negative result does not rule out an infection with vCJD.

Considering the epidemiological situation in Germany which is presently characterized by a prevalence and incidence too low to be measured, it is impossible in the current situation to quantify the increase of safety that is to be gained by screening for vCJD in terms of avoiding transfusion-transmitted vCJD.

6.2 Specificity

Up to now available investigations using very small sample numbers indicate an unsatisfactory specificity. With all due caution one has to assume a rate of false-positive results of approximately 2%. Only by extensive studies using samples from blood donors will it be possible to establish a test-immanent specificity of the various assays. The medico-legal difficulties involved have been discussed above under section 5.

On behalf of a maximal safety for transfusion recipients, all donations showing reactive screening results would have to be destroyed and actually, as a consequence in the absence of confirmation tests, donors would have to be excluded from further blood donation. Moreover, to be consistent, a look-back procedure would have to be initiated covering the entire donor history as far back as 1980, and recipients of blood products as well as the plasma fractionation industry would have to be notified. In Germany in 2006 4,595,484 homologous whole blood donations and 1,731,921 plasma and thrombocyte apheresis donations were collected [56]. On average, whole-blood donors donate every 6 months and apheresis donors once every month [2]. Based on an assumed rate of 2% false-positive results, at least in the first year after implementation of the test, approximately 92,000 whole-blood donors and up to 35,000 apheresis donors would have to be informed and excluded from further donations. Because repeat donors tend to donate regularly for years, the effort regarding look-back measures would be extraordinary. The same applies to apheresis donors who donate very frequently and to plasma donors whose plasma for fractionation is part of a plasma pool used for the manufacture of various plasma products.

6.3 Ethical Problems

Based on the actual epidemiological situation in Germany, it can be assumed that in fact almost none of the reactive results would indicate a real preclinical vCJD. If donors as well as recipients of blood products produced earlier were informed about a very vague suspicion concerning a fatal disease that can neither be ultimately ruled out nor treated, a considerable psychological strain for those concerned would be caused that might have conceivable respective consequences, potentially culminating in suicide.

Those concerned will ask a number of questions:

- When did the infection happen?
- How likely is my becoming ill?
- When will the disease break out, what are its symptoms?
- In case I was infectious, how can I transmit the agent?
- Do I have to inform my partner?
- Is a sexual transmission possible?
- May I become pregnant, and how high is the risk of transmission to the fetus?
- If my blood is infectious, what do I have to do if I suffer an injury?

Based on the current state of knowledge, one would give soothing answers, but this would be in stark contrast to the measures to be initiated for the sake of consistency.

Donors concerned (as well as recipients of blood components from these donors) would have to be advised to stop to donate blood, plasma, sperm, tissues or organs in the future. On the occasion of every medical, surgical and dental intervention they would have to inform about their existing potential infectivity. Medical institutions would have to implement considerably more measures than before to minimize the risk of these patients to transmit pathogenic prions. In the UK several hundred hemophiliacs had been treated with coagulation products that were possibly contaminated with the vCJD agent. Experiences from these persons in the UK showed that for example it had become very difficult for these patients to receive dental treatment.

Medical personnel with a reactive result in a vCJD test would have to stop performing certain parts of the job that are associated with a higher risk of injury (similar to those individuals infected with hepatitis B or hepatitis C).

Apart from family distress and depression, grave disadvantages must be taken into consideration, e.g. when contracting life insurance, vocational disability insurance or private health insurance, because of a diagnostic result which is highly likely to be false in diagnosing preclinical vCJD.

Apart from this, on implementing such diagnostic assays, adequately trained medical and pastoral personnel will have to be available to carry out information and counseling of the donors concerned, which is required in accordance with the TFG.

One way of overcoming this set of problems would be, on account of currently unreliable data, to generally not inform individuals about a reactive result on performing a vCJD test. However, if a vCJD case should actually be diagnosed later on, or even another person be infected or have been infected in the past, accusations of violating due diligence are to be expected.

On the other hand, the specifications of the TFG must be observed (see also section 5). A justifiable suspicion for an infection with vCJD based on the test results will initiate a look-back procedure in addition to destroying the actual donation. However, the donor has to be informed only after a confirmed diagnosis of a symptomatic disease or an infection, even though further donations will most probably become useless on account of their inherent albeit small risk. Furthermore, the donor is often suspended electronically and will be deferred without previous explanation, e.g. on the occasion of a computer-based mobile data entry. Under the present legal position in Germany, only if the donor actively requests an explanation of the reason for deferral, the blood service is allowed to extensively inform him/her about a justifiable suspicion.

In this situation, legally accepted definitions of both a justifiable suspicion and a confirmed diagnosis of vCJD must already be developed before performance evaluation and before, during and after implementation of a new diagnostic assay. These definitions are to be continuously updated according to the state of knowledge.

In order to establish definite rules for all concerned and to prevent subsequent criminal conviction, a consensus must be reached on the legal, political as well as social level regarding the resulting direct and indirect consequences and measures.

6.4 Restrictions on Supply

Based on an average frequency of donating whole blood of once every 6 months and of donating by apheresis of once every month [2] and also including the numbers mentioned under section 6.2, in 2006, approximately 2.3 million persons donated whole blood and 144,000 persons blood components or intermediates obtained by apheresis.

Assuming again the scenario of 2% false-positive results, in the first 12 months after test implementation, approximately 46,000 whole blood and 2,900 apheresis donations would be excluded from further blood donations. Thus the supply would be reduced by approximatley 92,000 erythrocyte concentrates and 23,000 l of plasma obtained from whole blood donations and approximately 35,000 blood components obtained by apheresis techniques. A further deterioration in supply is to be expected, especially regarding erythrocytes that at this stage have already begun to fail to meet demands.

Furthermore, it must be taken into consideration that 3 new donors have to be recruited within 12 months to replace 1 donor regularly donating whole blood [2]. To keep up the present supply, approximately 140,000 persons have to be newly motivated to donate blood.

In the context of the increasingly tight blood supply situation in Germany, a retraction of donors of the magnitude mentioned above would inevitably result in further bottleneck situations in supply, in the worst-case scenario leading to a collapsed service. This also applies in cases when an information of the donor is abandoned and just the respective donation is not released for use.

Deficits in plasma donations – and to a lesser extent in plasma for fractionation produced from whole blood – would lead to serious problems in supplying patients with immunoglobulins, coagulation factors, and other medical drugs produced from plasma. Whether imported plasma that was tested negative for vCJD became available for compensation is doubtful because donor retractions related to a test implementation would lead to a further shortage of plasma as a resource also on an international level.

6.5 *Feasibility*

Particularly for large blood services, it will only be possible to screen for prions if high-throughput automats are available. On account of the necessary release of blood components within 24 h or less after collection, the mere duration of the test should not be significantly longer than 4 h. It is impossible to delay the release for several days, especially for short-lived preparations like thrombocyte concentrates that, adapted for patients, have to be applied urgently or vitally important. Presently no suitable automated systems and corresponding reagents are available for these requirements. Until a minimum test specificity of 99.5% is reached for the assays (minimum requirement of the common technical specifications regarding infection serological assays), an implementation of an assay will be problematic as a result of the difficulties described in section 6.2. A specificity that is even higher would be preferable.
In addition, the legislator has to generate regulations permitting to test the feasibility and specificity of diagnostic assays available or under development under the conditions of a blood service, so that their viability can be assessed at all. Legal certainty must be established here about the fact that an information of the donors, as well as consequences for the release of blood donations or look-back procedures and ultimately the recall of donations, may be abandoned if test results are indeterminate. This implies to deliberately run the risk of the highly improbable case, which however cannot be completely ruled out, that a reactive result is indeed attributable to preclinical vCJD which may become conspicuous only after months or even years.
On account of previously applied technology and technical equipment requirements, a longer period of transition is needed before nationwide screening can be implemented, because probably methods have to be implemented that have never been used routinely in the blood services. This transition period will also be necessary to arrange for the required investments, computer-based support and quality management/validation of the diagnostic assays.

6.6 *Costs*

At present no estimation can be made regarding supplementary costs for investments, reagents, and personnel required.

6.7 *Quality Management*

On account of the rareness of the disease, it is not possible at present to provide suitable samples for external quality assurance. There are no independent positive or negative controls. Thus, it is not possible to compare results of different tests. Accordingly, a validation by the user is only possible in terms of a performance evaluation. Therefore, the establishment of appropriate conditions should be aimed for. For example, every diagnostic assay to be implemented should be evaluated with an independent panel of human blood samples from patients with different TSE isoforms and other neurodegenerative diseases as well as from healthy controls.

6.8 *Safety Considerations*

According to the type of assay selected, safety precautions have to be taken that largely prevent hazards for the personnel. This applies especially to techniques which potentially generate pathological PrPs. In that case in every institution performing such tests a BSL-3 laboratory is required with the corresponding investment and maintenance costs.

6.9 *Availability*

On implementation of screening tests for prions in blood donations, it has to be ensured that manufacturing capacities of the companies in question are sufficiently large to guarantee an uninterrupted supply with test kits of consistent quality. The same is true for technical support. To interrupt the screening after it was implemented because of unavailable test kits would also be precarious for ethical reasons. Because different approaches will probably be used in the assays, a short-term switch-over to instruments and reagents from other manufacturers will be almost impossible.

7 Conclusion and Assessment

The disease vCJD is definitely fatal according to the current state of knowledge and is transmissible by blood transfusion. To prevent transmission of vCJD by blood transfusion and to protect transfusion recipients, the existence of a suitable screening assay for vCJD in blood donors would be very valuable. Still in 2006 the last report of the Working Group came to the following conclusion: 'No such test is currently available nor is its availability foreseeable. Providing resources for developing suitable test methods should therefore be treated with high priority' [2]. This situation has changed in the meantime.
The detection of the pathological PrP^{TSE} has to be very sensitive and simultaneously specific in a background of physiological PrP^{C} present in a concentration that is several magnitudes

higher. The amino acid sequence of PrP^C is identical to that of PrP^{TSE} but is simply folded differently. Therefore, high demands are made on the methods. At present there are various far advanced assays under development, so that it is only a question of time when the first screening assays for vCJD will be offered and marketed. At present, in accordance with the applicable IVD law, it would be rather simple for the manufacturers to obtain the CE marking for such assays and thus make them marketable. A formal application to the European Commission is required in order to include new diagnostic assays into list A ('high-risk products'). Such an application has been filed but might still take some time. This process should be emphatically supported.

The mandatory verification and validation of such assays is especially difficult for technical reasons because suitable vCJD-positive samples are very scarce. Therefore, it is suggested to support the creation of suitable sample panels. Such panels should predominantly contain samples from patients with various TSE isoforms and with dementia of other etiologies as well as from healthy controls.

Provided that they are technically safe and suitable, IVDs for the detection of infections causing severe diseases like vCJD have to be employed in assessing the fitness of a blood donor in accordance with the TFG. This emphasizes the necessity of a performance evaluation study for such novel assays regarding their suitability and safety. After successful admission into list A of the IVD guideline [54], the performance of the assay must be tested in test persons and patients. A precondition for the performance evaluation study of an IVD for the detection of vCJD infections in blood donors is the informed consent of the participants. Participants in a study are entitled at any time to learn their test results and would have to receive suitable counseling in case the test was reactive. The ethics boards involved are also called upon extensively in designing such studies. The main issue is that by a reactive test result a seemingly healthy person would be put under suspicion of the imminent outbreak of a fatal disease for which the latency is unknown and that cannot be treated at this point, while confirmation assays to clarify this suspected diagnosis are lacking at present.

Similar ethical problems would result on implementation of such assays for routine screening of blood donors. A positive test result would imply the obligation of the physician responsible to inform the donor about this fact and to give advice, in case the assay was assumed to be reliable and suitable to detect a vCJD infection. Already in the case of a 'justifiable suspicion' that a donor was infected with vCJD, the physician responsible is obligated to eliminate the donation, to trace and inform as well as examine any recipients, and to notify the competent authorities, unless there is a reasonable assumption of its probably being a false-positive result. In the context of this, but also regarding the necessary performance evaluation of the diagnostic assays, guidelines for the information of donors and recipients have to be developed. On the part of the blood services involved, there is an enormous desire for legal security.

In principle, the current development of screening assays for the detection of vCJD is welcome. However, before such assays can be marketed and put to routine use, there remain considerable problems. In view of the presently known epidemiological situation of vCJD in Germany, in view of only four confirmed transmissions by blood transfusion in the UK, and in view of the difficulties described above regarding performance evaluation, the implementation of vCJD diagnostic assays appears to be inadvisable at present.

Members of the Working Group

Michael Beekes, Robert Koch-Institut, Berlin
Johannes Blümel, Paul-Ehrlich-Institut, Langen
Reinhard Burger, Robert Koch-Institut, Berlin
Christian von Dewitz, State Office of Health and Social Affairs (LaGeSo), Berlin
Albrecht Gröner, CSL Behring, Marburg
Margarethe Heiden, Paul-Ehrlich-Institut, Langen
Hans Kretzschmar, Institute of Neuropathology and Prion Research, Ludwig-Maximilians-University Munich
Micha Nübling, Paul-Ehrlich-Institut, Langen
Uwe Schlenkrich, German Hemophilia Society (DHG), Hamburg
Volkmar Schottstedt, Blood Services of the German Red Cross West (DRK), Hagen
Rainer Seitz (central coordination), Paul-Ehrlich-Institut, Langen
Johanna Strobel, Federal Ministry of Health, Bonn
Hannelore Willkommen, NewLab BioQuality GmbH, Regulatory Affairs and Biological Safety Consulting, Erkrath
Carl-Heinz Wirsing von König, HELIOS Clinical Center, Krefeld
Inga Zerr, National Reference Center for the Surveillance of TSE, University Clinical Center, Göttingen

The members of the Working Group were appointed by the German Federal Minister of Health.

References

1 Joint press release of the Paul-Ehrlich-Institut and the Robert Koch-Institut. Gesamtstrategie Blutversorgung im Angesicht der BSE-Krise. *www.pei.de/cln_115/nn_157198/DE/infos/presse/pm/archiv/2001/14.html.*

2 Working Group 'Overall Blood Supply with Regard to Variant Creutzfeldt-Jakob Disease (vCJD)': Overall Blood Supply with Regard to Variant Creutzfeldt-Jakob Disease (vCJD) – Report of the Working Group Commissioned by the German Federal Ministry of Health, April 13, 2006 (Update of the Report from August 17, 2001). Transfus Med Hemother 2006:33(suppl 2).

3 Seitz R, von Auer F, Blümel J, Burger R, Buschmann A, Dietz K, Heiden M, Hitzler WE, Klamm H, Kreil T, Kretzschmar H, Nübling M, Offergeld R, Pauli G, Schottstedt V, Volkers P, Zerr I: Impact of vCJD on blood supply. Biologicals 2007;35:79–97.

4 Creutzfeldt HG: Über eine eigenartige herdförmige Erkrankung des Zentralnervensystems. Z Ges Neurol Psychiatr 1920;57:1–18.

5 Jakob A: Über eigenartige Erkrankungen des Zentralnervensystems mit bemerkenswertem anatomischem Befund (Spastische Pseudosklerose – Encephalomyelopathie mit disseminierten Degenerationsherden). Dtsch Z Nervenheilk 1921;70: 132–146.

6 Glatzel M, Abela E, Maissen M, Aguzzi A: Extraneural pathogenic prion protein in sporadic Creutzfeldt-Jakob disease. N Engl J Med 2003;349: 1812–1820.

7 Bishop MT, Ritchie DL, Will RG, Ironside JW, Head MW, Thomson V, Bruce M, Manson JC: No major change in vCJD agent strain after secondary transmission via blood transfusion. PLoS ONE 2008;3: 1–6.

8 The National Creutzfeldt-Jakob Disease Surveillance Unit (NCJDSU): Variant Creutzfeldt-Jakob Disease. Current data. *www.cjd.ed.ac.uk/vcjdworld.htm.*

9 Dietz K, Raddatz G, Wallis J, Müller N, Zerr I, Duerr H-P, Lefèvre H, Seifried E, Löwer J:. Blood transfusion and spread of variant Creutzfeldt-Jakob disease. Emerg Infect Dis 2007;13:89–96.
10 Clarke P, Will RG, Ghani AC: Is there the potential for an epidemic of variant Creutzfeldt-Jakob disease via blood transfusion in the UK? J R Soc Interface 2007;4:675–684.
11 Garske T: Presentation at the Paul-Ehrlich-Institut on May 28, 2008.
12 Mead S, Joiner S, Desbruslais M, Beck JA, O'Donoghue M, Lantos P, Wadsworth JDF, Collinge J: Creutzfeldt-Jakob disease, prion protein gene codon 129VV, and a novel PrPSc type in a young British woman. Arch Neurol 2007;64: 1780–1784.
13 Coghlan A: Mysterious death reignites vCJD fears. NewScientist 2008;2637:11.
14 Gambetti P, Dong Z, Yuan J, et al: A novel human disease with abnormal prion protein sensitive to protease. Ann Neurol 2008;63:697–708.
15 Krebs B, Bader B, Klehmet J, Grasbon-Frodl E, Oertel WH, Zerr I, Stricker S, Zschenderlein R, Kretzschmar HA: A novel subtype of Creutzfeldt–Jakob disease characterized by a small 6 kDa PrP fragment. Acta Neuropathol 2007;114:195–199.
16 Parchi P, Giese A; Capellari S, Brown P, Schulz-Schaeffer W, Windl O, Zerr I, Budka H, Kopp N, Piccardo P, Poser S, Rojiani A, Streichemberger N, Julien J, Vital C, Ghetti B, Gambetti P, Kretzschmar H: Classification of sporadic Creutzfeldt-Jakob disease based on molecular and phenotypic analysis of 300 subjects. Ann Neurol 1999;46:224–233.
17 Oesch B, Westaway D, Wälchli M, McKinley MP, Kent SBH, Aebersold R, Barry RA, Tempst P, Teplow DB, Hood LE, Prusiner SB, Weissmann C: A cellular gene encodes scrapie PrP(27–30) protein. Cell 1985;40:735–746.
18 Basler K, Oesch B, Scott M, Westaway D, Wälchli M, Groth DF, McKinley MP, Prusiner SB, Weissmann C: Scrapie and cellular PrP isoforms are encoded by the same chromosomal gen. Cell 1986;46: 417–428.
19 Caughey BW, Dong A, Bhat KS, Ernst D, Hayes SF, Caughey WS: Secondary structure analysis of the scrapie-associated protein PrP(27-30) in water by infrared spectroscopy. Biochemistry 1991;30: 7672–7680.
20 Pan KM, Baldwin M, Nguyen J, Gasset M, Serban A, Groth D, Mehlhorn I, Huang Z, Fletterick RJ, Cohen FE, Prusiner SB: Conversion of alpha-helices into beta-sheets features the formation of the scrapie prion proteins. Proc Natl Acac Sci U S A 1993;90: 10962–10966.
21 Safar J, Wille H, Itri V, Groth D, Serban H, Torchia M, Cohen FE, Prusiner SB: Eight prion strains have PrPSc molecules with different conformations. Nat Med 1998;4:1157–1165.
22 Kascsak RJ, Rubenstein R, Merz PA, Tonna-DeMasi M, Fersko R, Carp RI, Wisniewski HM, Diringer H: Mouse polyclonal and monoclonal antibody to scrapie-associated fibril proteins. J Virol 1987;61:3688–3693.
23 Barry RA, Prusiner SB: Monoclonal antibodies to the cellular and scrapie prion protein. J Infect Dis 1986; 154:518–521.
24 Korth C, Stierli B, Streit P, Moser M, Schaller O, Fischer R, Schulz-Schaeffer W, Kretzschmar H, Raeber A, Braun U, Ehrensperger F, Hornemann S, Glucksbuber R, Rick R, Billeter M, Wüthrich K, Oesch B: Prion (PrPSc)-specific epitope defined by a monoclonal antibody. Nature 1997;390:74–77.
25 Moroncini G, Mangieri M, Morbin M, Mazzoleni G, Ghetti B, Gabrielli A, Williamson RA, Giaccone G, Tagliavini F: Pathogenic prion protein is specifically recognized in situ by a novel PrP conformational antibody. Neurobiol Dis 2006;23:717–724.
26 Ulrih NP, Skrt M, Veranic P, Galvani V, Vranac T, Curin Serbec V: Oligomeric forms of peptide fragments PrP(214-226) in solution are preferentially recognized by PrPSc-specific antibody. Biochem Biophys Res Commun 2006;344:1320–1326.
27 Salguero FJ, Diaz-San Segundo F, Brun A, Cano MJ, Torres JM: Comparison of three monoclonal antibodies for use in immunohistochemical detection of bovine spongiform encephalopathy protease-resistant prion protein. J Vet Diagn Invest 2006;18: 106–109.
28 Biasini E, Seegulam ME, Patti BN, Solforosi L, Medrano AZ, Christensen HM, Senatore A, Chiesa R, Williamson RA, Harris DA: Non-infectious aggregates of the prion protein react with several PrPSc-directed antibodies. J Neurochem 2008;105: 2190–2204.
29 Morel N, Simion S, Frobert Y, Volland H, Mourton-Gilles C, Negro A, Sorgato MC, Creminon C, Grassi J: Selective and efficient immunoprecipitation of the disease-associated form of the prion protein can be mediated by non-specific interactions between monoclonal antibodies and scrapie-associated fibrils. J Biochem Chem 2004;279:30143–30149.
30 Pan T, Li R, Wong B-S, Kang S-C, Ironside J, Sy M-S: Novel antibody-lectin enzyme-linked immunosorbent assay that distinguishes prion proteins in sporadic and variant cases of Creutzfeldt-Jakob disease. J Clin Microbiol 2005;43:1118–1126.
31 Safar JG, Geschwind MD, Deering C, Didorenko S, Sattavat M, Sanchez H, Serban A, Vey M, Baron H, Giles K, Miller BL, DeArmond SJ: Diagnosis of human prion disease. Proc Natl Acad Si U S A 2005; 102:3501–3506.
32 Bessen RA, Marsh RF: Biochemical and physical properties of the prion protein from two strains of the transmissible mink encephalopathy agent. J Virol 1992;66:2096–2101.
33 Barron RM, Campbell SL, King D, Bellon A, Chapman KE, Williamson RA, Manson JC: High titers of transmissible spongiform encephalopathy infectivity associated with extremly low levels of PrPSc in vivo. J Biol Chem 2007;282:35878–35886.
34 Berardi VA, Cardone F, Valanzano A, Lu M, Pocchiari M: Preparation of soluble infectious samples from scrapie-infected brain: new tool to study the clearance of transmissible spongiform encephalopathy agents during plasma fractionation. Transfusion 2006; 46:652–658.
35 Wadsworth JDF, Joiner S, Hill AF, Campbell TA, Desbruslais M, Luthert PJ, Collinge J: Tissue distribution of protein resistant prion protein in variant Creutzfeldt-Jakob disease using a highly sensitive immunoblotting assay. Lancet 2001;358:171–180.
36 Silveira JR, Raymond GJ, Hughson AG, Race RE, Sim VL, Hayes SF, Caughey B: The most infectious prion protein particle. Nature 2005;437:257–261.
37 Brown P, Rohwer RG, Dunstan BC, MacAuley C, Gajdusek DC, Drohan WN: The distribution of infectivity in blood components and plasma derivatives in experimental models of transmissible spongiform encephalopathy. Transfusion 1998;38:810–816.
38 Brown P, Cervenáková L, McShane LM, Barber P, Rubenstein R, Drohan WN: Further studies of blood infectivity in an experimental model of transmissible spongiform encephalopathy, with an explanation of why blood components do not transmit Creutzfeldt-Jakob disease in humans. Transfusion 1999;39:1169–1178.
39 Cervenáková L, Yakovleva O, McKenzie C, Kolchinski S, McShane L, Drohan WN, Brown P: Similar levels of infectivity in the blood of mice infected with human-derived vCJD and GSS strains of transmissible spongiform encephalopathy. Transfusion 2003;43:1687–1694.
40 Houston F, Foster JD, Chong A, Hunter N, Bostock CJ: Transmission of BSE by blood transfusion in sheep. Lancet 2000;356:999–1000.
41 Hunter N, Foster J, Chong A, McCutcheon S, Parnham D, Eaton S, MacKenzie C, Houston F: Transmission of prion diseases by blood transfusion. J Gen Virol 2002;83:2897–2905.
42 Yakovleva O, Janiak A, McKenzie C, McShane L, Brown P, Cervenáková L: Effect of protease treatment on plasma infectivity in variant Creutzfeldt-Jakob disease mice. Transfusion 2004;44:1700–1705.
43 Minor P: NIBSC, presentation at the workshop of the European Commission on 26 October 2007 in Brussels.
44 Uger M: Amorfix Life Sciences, presentation at the workshop of the European Commission on 26 October 2007 in Brussels.
45 Health Protection Agency: TED-Publication 30072–2007, February 6, 2007.
46 Pan T, Sethi J, Nelsen C, Rudolph A, Cervenáková L, Brown P, Orser CS: Detection of misfolded prion protein in blood with conformationally sensitive peptides. Transfusion 2007;47:1418–1425.
47 Saborio GP, Permanne B, Soto C: Sensitive detection of pathological prion protein by cyclic amplification of protein misfolding. Nature 2001;411: 810–813.
48 Atarashi R, Moore RA, Sim VL, Hughson AG, Dorward DW, Onwubiko HA, Priola SA, Caughey B: Ultrasensitive detection of scrapie prion protein using seeded conversion of recombinant prion protein. Nat Methods 2007;4:645–650.
49 Atarashi R, Wilham JM, Christensen L, Hughson AG, Moore RA, Johnson LM, Onwubiko HA, Priola SA, Caughey B: Simplified ultrasensitive prion detection by recombinant PrP conversion with shaking. Nat Methods 2008;5:211–212;
50 Colby DW, Zhang Q, Wang S, Groth D, Legname G, Riesner D, Prusiner SB: Prion detection by an amyloid seeding assay. Proc Natl Acad Sci U S A 2007;104:20914–20919.
51 Mahal SP, Baker CA, Demczyk CA, Smith EW, Julius C, Weissmann C: Prion strain discrimination in cell culture: the cell panel assay. Proc Natl Acad Sci U S A 2007;104:20908–20913.
52 Falsig J, Julius C, Margalith I, Schwarz P, Heppner FL, Aguzzi A: A versatile prion replication assay in organotypic brain slices. Nat Neurosci 2008;11: 109–117.
53 Fagge TJ, Barclay GR, Stove GC, Stove G, Robinson MJ, Head MW, Ironside JW, Turner ML: Application of atomic dielectric resonance spectroscopy for the screening of blood samples from patients with clinical variant and sporadic CJD. J Transl Med 2007;5:41.
54 Directive 98/79/EG of the European Parliament and of the Council of 27 October 1998 on in vitro diagnostic medical devices. Official Journal of the European Communities L 331/1 of December 7, 1998.
55 Amorfix: Press Release of August 19, 2008.
56 Haschberger B, Henseler O, Hesse J, Heiden M, Seitz R: Bericht zur Meldung nach § 21 TFG für die Jahre 2005 und 2006. Bundesgesundheitsbl Gesundheitsforsch Gesundheitsschutz 2008;51:353–372.

Mannheimer Transfusionsgespräche 2009
(ehemals Marburger Transfusionsgespräche)

Praktische Probleme und aktuelle Themen in der Transfusionsmedizin - Erfahrungsaustausch zwischen Transfusionsmedizinern, Transfusionsverantwortlichen und –beauftragten sowie Qualitätsbeauftragten

27. und 28. Februar 2009, Mannheim
Fortbildungspunkte der LÄK Baden Württemberg

Universitätsklinikum Mannheim, Die **Alte Brauerei**, Käfertaler Straße 162, Mannheim

---

Der Hauptveranstaltung der «Mannheimer Transfusionsgespräche» wird der
«2. Erfahrungsaustausch für Qualitätsbeauftragte Hämotherapie»
27. Februar 2009 vormittags von 9.00-12.00 Uhr vorangestellt
Leitung Dr. R. Kaiser, LÄK Hessen und
Prof. (em) Dr. V. Kretschmer (IAKH e. V.)
Keine Teilnahmegebühr, jedoch Extraanmeldung erforderlich. Anmeldung und weitere Infos bei der LÄK Hessen: Tel.: 069/97672-195, E-Mail: qs@laekh.de; www.laekh.de

---

Mannheimer Transfusionsgespräche, 27. und 28. Februar 2009
27. Februar 2009, 13.00-18.30 Uhr
28. Februar 2009, 8.30-15.30 Uhr

Avisierte Themen:

- Bereitstellung von Blutkonserven
- Schätzung des chirurgischen Blutverlustes
- Transfusionsbedarf und Demografie
- Meldepflichten
- Fehlerregister der IAKH
- Radiofrequenzidentifikation von Blutkonserven
- Chronische Anämie – Erkennung und Therapie in verschiedenen Fachgebieten
- Erythropoetin-Therapie
- Transfusion in der Geburtshilfe: Placento-fetale Transfusion – irreguläre Antikörper – Frühgeborenen-Transfusion
- Massivtransfusion
- Die neuen Querschnitts-Leitlinien zur Hämotherapie/Logistik der Thrombozyten-Transfusion
- Aktuelles

Die genauen Themen und Referenten werden aus Gründen der Aktualität kurzfristig festgelegt und über Internet bekannt gegeben. Aktuelle Informationen zu den Veranstaltungen und Anmeldeformular unter: www.IAKH.de

Teilnahmegebühren bis zum 15.02.2009 (danach 20% Aufschlag):
Euro 20,- für IAKH-Mitglieder (24,-€), 30,-- für Nichtmitglieder (36,--€)
Freitagabend Abendessen 15,-- € / pro Person (Extraanmeldung erforderlich)
Bezahlung bitte auf das Seminarkonto der IAKH e. V.:
Interdisziplinäre ARGE f. Klinische Hämotherapie e. V.
Konto-Nr:46 57 90 11, BLZ: 513 900 00, Volksbank Mittelhessen eG
Stichwort: „Mannheimer Transfusionsgespräche"

Anmeldung/ Themenvorschläge:
Fax: +49 64 21/58 6 54 95 E-Mail: iakh-kongress@iakh.de oder
E-Mail: Thoms.Frietsch@med.uni-marburg.de
Prof. Dr. Thomas Frietsch,
Klinik für Anästhesie und Intensivtherapie, Universitätsklinikum Giessen und Marburg GmbH, Standort Marburg, Baldingerstraße, 35043 Marburg

Neues raumtemperaturstabiles NovoSeven®: Mehr Therapiekomfort für Hämophilie-Patienten

NovoSeven®, das einzige rekombinante aktivierte Faktor-VII-Produkt (rFVIIa) zur Behandlung von Blutungsepisoden bei Patienten mit Hemmkörper-Hämophilie, liegt ab Februar 2009 als raumtemperaturstabile Formulierung vor. Dies gab das Unternehmen Novo Nordisk Pharma GmbH bekannt. Das Präparat ist dadurch jederzeit verfügbar und ermöglicht eine sofortige Behandlung von Blutungen. Dies bedeutet einen erhöhten Therapiekomfort und damit eine deutliche Verbesserung der Lebensqualität für die Patienten. Die neue raumtemperaturstabile Formulierung von NovoSeven® bietet den Vorteil, dass sie jederzeit verfügbar ist. Dies gibt dem Patienten die Möglichkeit, NovoSeven® im Fall einer Blutung jederzeit – auch unterwegs – rasch und effektiv anwenden zu können. Die raumtemperaturstabile Formulierung ersetzt die bisherige Formulierung von NovoSeven®. Das raumtemperaturstabile NovoSeven® ist bei Raumtemperatur (bis zu 25°C) bis zu 2 Jahre stabil [1]. Das neue Präparat ist bioäquivalent und besitzt vergleichbare pharmakokinetische Eigenschaften wie die Vorgängerformulierung [2]. Da die Konzentration der rekonstituierten Lösung bei der raumtemperaturstabilen Formulierung im Vergleich zur Vorgänger-Formulierung erhöht ist, ist das Injektionsvolumen bei dem neuen Präparat um 40% reduziert. Ein weiterer Vorteil: Die Berechnung des Injektionsvolumens wird erleichtert, da das neue rFVIIa-Präparat nun in ganzzahligen Dosisstärken von 1, 2 und 5 mg vorliegt. Zu dem raumtemperaturstabilen NovoSeven®-Präparat gibt es zusätzlich eine tragbare, stabile Reise-Box, in der alle Utensilien für die Behandlung einer einzelnen Blutung unterwegs zur Verfügung stehen. Die Raumtemperaturstabilität ermöglicht einen sofortigen Therapiebeginn, sodass Blutungen schnell gestoppt werden können [3].

Referenzen

1 NovoSeven® (1 mg (50 kIE)/2 mg (100 kIE)/5 mg (250 kIE)) Fachinformation, Stand: September 2008.
2 Bysted BV et al: Haemophilia 2007;13:527–532.
3 Lusher JM. Blood Coagul Fibrinolysis 2000;11(Suppl 1):45–49.

Weitere Informationen bei
Medizin & Markt GmbH
Franziska Wagenschwanz
Schackstraße 1/IV, 80539 München
Tel.+49 89 383930-22, Fax +49 89 339075
wagenschwanz@medizin-und-markt.de

Erstmals interaktiver Workshop zur Hämophilie-Therapie: Frühe Behandlung entscheidend

Eine frühe prophylaktische Therapie mit dem fehlenden Gerinnungsfaktor kann das Hemmkörperrisiko sowie die Anzahl der Blutungen bei Hämophilie-Patienten deutlich reduzieren. Dies zeigen Studiendaten [1, 2], die auf einem interaktiven Computer-gestützten Workshop von Wyeth zur Hämophilietherapie in Berlin vorgestellt wurden. Ein weiterer wichtiger Aspekt des Workshops war die Bedeutung der Publikation neuer Daten in der Hämophilie. Gemeinsamer Konsens von jungen und erfahrenen Hämophilie-Behandlern beim Workshop: Um langfristig die Hämophilietherapie weiter zu optimieren, sollten Pharmakovigilanz-Untersuchungen und andere Erhebungen unterstützt werden. Für die rekombinanten Produkte ReFacto® (Moroctocog alfa) und BeneFIX® (Nonacog alfa) von Wyeth gibt es bereits solche nicht-interventionellen Studien.

Der 2-tätige Workshop fand in diesem Jahr erstmals in dieser Form statt und wurde von der Ärztekammer Berlin mit 10 CME-Punkten zertifiziert. Aufgegriffen wurden verschiedene Aspekte der Hämophilietherapie sowie Herausforderungen des Praxisalltags in Vorträgen und interaktiven Falldiskussionen. In der 2-tägigen Veranstaltung trugen insgesamt 17 Referenten dazu bei, in Frontalvorträgen verschiedene Themenblöcke der Hämophilie zu beleuchten. Die anschließenden interaktiven Falldiskussionen mit TED-Abstimmung förderten die fachliche Diskussion und einen regen Austausch unter den Experten. Der Workshop fand in diesem Jahr erstmals in dieser Computer-gestützten Form statt, soll aber auch interaktiv fortgeführt werden.

Referenzen

1 Gouw S, van der Bom J, van den Berg: Treatment-related risk factors of inhibitor development in previously untreated patients with hemophilia A: The CANAL cohort study. Blood 2007;109:4648–4654.
2 Manco-Johnson M et al.: Prophylaxis versus episodic treatment to prevent joint disease in boys with severe hemophilia. N Engl J Med 2007;357:535–54.

Weitere Informationen bei
Wyeth Pharma GmbH
Pressestelle, Mirja Kaupmann
Wienburgstraße 207, 48159 Münster
Tel.+49 251 204-1226, Fax -2033
www.wyeth.de

Ticker+++ Ticker+++ Ticker+++ Ticker+++ Ticker+++ Ticker+++ Ticker+++

Leo Pharma GmbH. Tumorpatienten haben ein überproportional erhöhtes Risiko für venöse Thromboembolien (VTE). Fachgesellschaften empfehlen deshalb zur perioperativen Thromboseprophylaxe und zur medikamentösen Langzeittherapie nach einer VTE den Einsatz eines niedermolekularen Heparins. Mittel der Wahl bei diesen Risikopatienten ist Tinzaparin (innohep®).

Wefra PR Gesellschaft für Public Relations mbH
Judith Schönberger
Tel. +49 69 695008-76
js@wefra.de

Mundipharma GmbH. Als First-line-Therapie von indolenten NHL und Mantelzell-Lymphomen war Bendamustin + Rituximab (BR) in einer Studie ebenso effektiv wie CHOP-R, bei besserer Verträglichkeit. Die Phase-II-Studie CLL2M untersuchte BR auch bei rezidivierter/refraktärer und unvorbehandelter CLL. Um den Stellenwert von BR als First-line-Therapie der CLL weiter zu definieren, wird es nun mit Fludarabin + Cyclophosphamid + Rituximab (FCR) verglichen (Studie CLL10).

POMME-med GmbH
Dr.Petra Ortner
ortner@pomme-med.de

Alexion Pharma Germany GmbH. Der rekombinante monoklonale Antikörper Soliris® (Eculizumab) greift kausal in den Pathomechanismus der paroxysmalen nächtlichen Hämoglobinurie (PNH) ein. Die Erkrankung führt zu einem erhöhten Risiko für lebensbedrohliche thromboembolische Komplikationen. Mit der deutlichen Verbesserung der Beschwerden und der Reduktion von thromboembolischen Ereignissen hat Eculizumab den Verlauf der PNH maßgeblich verändert und neue Maßstäbe für die Behandlung gesetzt.

Alexion Pharma Germany GmbH
Melanie Hansen
hansenm@alxn.com

KARGER
Fax + 49 761 4 52 07 14
information@karger.de
www.karger.com

Transfusion Medicine and Hemotherapy

Meetings and Conferences · Tagungen und Kongresse

Transfus Med Hemother 2009;36:96

04.02.–07.02.2009 **Wien** Österreich	**GTH 2009 – 53rd Annual Meeting Society of Thrombosis and Haemostasis Research**	**Auskunft:** Mondial Congress & Events, Operngasse 20b, 1040 Wien, Österreich, Tel. 49 1 588 040 Gth2009@mondial-congress.com, www.gth2009.org
25.02.–27.02.2009 **Rom** Italien	**11th European Haemovigliance Seminar**	**Auskunft:** Eurocongress International Jan van Goyenkade 11 1075 HP Amsterdam, The Netherlands Tel. +31 20 679 3411 ehs@eurocongress.com www.eurocongress.com
27.02.–28.02.2009 **Mannheim** Deutschland	**8. IAKH Transfusions- und Hämotherapietage + Workshop für Qualitätsbeauftragte (ehemals «Marburger Transfusionsgespräche»)**	**Auskunft:** www.iakh.de
29.03.–01.04.2009 **Göteborg** Schweden	**EBTM 2009**	**Auskunft:** www.akm.ch/ebmt2009/
09.05.–12.05.2009 **Leipzig** Deutschland	**Deutscher Anästhesiecongress 2009**	**Auskunft:** MCN Medizinische Congressorganisation Nürnberg AG Neuwieder Str. 9, 90411 Nürnberg Tel. +49 911 39 31 60 mcn@mcn-nuernberg.de www.mcn-nuernberg.de
26.05.–27.05.2009 **Brüssel** Belgien	**The IPFA & PEI 16th Workshop on «Surveillance and Screening of Blood Borne Pathogens»**	**Auskunft:** IPFA, Plesmanlaan 125 1066 CX Amsterdam, The Netherlands Tel.: +31 20 512 3561 Fax +31 20 512 3559 ipfa@sanquin.nl www.ipfa.nl
04.06.–07.06.2009 **Berlin** Deutschland	**14th Congress of the European Hematology Association**	**Auskunft:** www.ehaweb.org
11.07.–17.07.2009 **Boston** USA	**XXII. Congress of the International Society on Thrombosis and Haemostasis**	**Auskunft:** www.isth2009.com Isth2009@mci-group.com
15.09.–18.09.2009 **Rostock** Deutschland	**42. Jahreskongress der Deutschen Gesellschaft für Transfusionsmedizin und Immunhämatologie (DGTI)**	**Auskunft:** Kongress- und Messebüro Lentzsch GmbH Seifgrundstraße 2, 61348 Bad Homburg Tel. +49 6172 6796-0, Fax -26 info@kmb-lentzsch.de, www.dgti.de
24.10.–27.10.2009 **New Orleans, LA** USA	**AABB Annual Meeting and TXPO 2009**	**Auskunft:** www.aabb.org
26.06.–01.07.2010 **Berlin** Deutschland	**XXXIst International Congress of the ISBT + 43. Jahreskongress der Deutschen Gesellschaft für Transfusionsmedizin und Immunhämatologie (DGTI)**	**Auskunft:** www.isbt-web.org oder Kongress- und Messebüro Lentzsch GmbH Seifgrundstraße 2, 61348 Bad Homburg Tel. +49 6172 6796-0, Fax -26 info@kmb-lentzsch.de, www.dgti.de
06.07.–10.07.2010 **Mailand** Italien	**21st Congress on Thrombosis**	**Auskunft:** www.thrombosis2010.org

KARGER

Fax +49 761 4 52 07 14
Information@Karger.de
www.karger.com

Accessible online at:
www.karger.com/tmh

Transfusion Medicine and Hemotherapy

Guidelines for Authors

Transfus Med Hemother 2009;36

Submission

TRANSFUSION MEDICINE AND HEMOTHERAPY is a peer-reviewed journal intended to provide a forum for presentation of all aspects of transfusion medicine, hemostaseology, and immunohematology. The journal publishes articles concerning scientific, technical and administrative aspects of blood banking, blood infusion, infusion therapy, and transplantation.

Manuscripts can now be submitted online: www.karger.com/tmh

Should you have any problems with electronic submission, or feel the need to submit the paper in a non-electronic form, please send your manuscript to:

S. Karger Verlag für Medizin und Naturwissenschaften GmbH
Attn.: Dr. Sven Riestenpatt
P.O. Box
79095 Freiburg (Germany)
Tel. +49 761 4520 722
Fax +49 761 4520 714
E-mail s.riestenpatt@karger.de

Language

All contributions (except for Commentaries and Congress Reports) must be written in English (American or British spelling and grammar).

Types of Papers and Allotted Number of Pages

Please print the manuscript 1 1/2-spaced with 3-cm margins (left and right). Use only one format (normal) for the document.

The text (including the summary) should be limited to the following number of pages:

	Printed pages	Equals approx. manuscript pages*
Review Article, Original Article	10	30
Case Report	3	9
Quality Management, Clinical Information	5	15
Letter to the Editor	2	6
Others	2	6

*** including title page, summary, illustrations, tables, and references.**
Each additional complete or partial page to print will be charged to the author.

Conditions

Acceptance of a manuscript is based on the evaluation by several reviewers (peer review).
Manuscripts are received with the explicit understanding that they are not under simultaneous consideration by any other publication. Submission of an article for publication implies the transfer of the copyright from the author to the publisher upon acceptance.
Once the manuscript is accepted for publication, all usage rights will be retained by the publisher. The assignment of usage rights applies to all print media as well as electronic offline and online media, including the Internet and data bases/data carriers of any kind. Accepted papers, in whole or in part, may not be translated into other languages, or reproduced by any mechanical or electronic means (including photocopying, recording and microcopying), or stored in a retrieval system without the written consent of the publisher.
It is the authors' responsibility to obtain permission to produce illustrations, tables, etc. from other publications.
All forms of support, including that from drug companies, and any potential source of conflict of interest should be acknowledged in the cover letter to the editor. Should the manuscript be accepted, the editor will discuss the extent of disclosure appropriate for publication with the authors.
The publisher reserves the right to edit the manuscript and decide on the layout.

Ethical and Legal Prerequisites

Manuscripts involving examinations of human subjects must include a statement that the trial protocol has been approved by an ethical committee and thus meets the standards of the Declaration of Helsinki in its revised version of 1975 and its amendments of 1983, 1989, and 1996 [JAMA 1997;277:925–926]. Accordingly, the subject's informed consent has to be mentioned in the manuscript. Information suitable to reveal the subject's identity is to be avoided.

Arrangement

Authors' affiliations and address of correspondence: Each author's full name, followed by their affiliation (hospital, institute etc. where the work was conducted) and the exact postal address of the corresponding author complete with postal code must be given. Please also supply phone and fax numbers, as well as e-mail address.

Title page: The first page of each paper should indicate the title (German and English) and a short title for use as running head.

Key Words: For indexing purposes, a list of 3–5 key words in English and German is essential. Whenever possible, use key words such as found in the Medical Subject Headings List (MeSH) of Index Medicus.

Summary: Summaries must be submitted in German and English. They must not exceed 200 words each. Summaries of Original Articles and Case Reports should be structured as follows: Background, Patients and Methods (or Material and Methods), Results, Conclusion.

Footnotes: Footnotes should be used only for tables.

Registered Trade Names: When first mentioned, registered trade names must be marked with the superscript registration symbol ® or ™. It is the sole responsibility of the author to ensure that this rule is followed properly.

Tables and Illustrations: Tables and illustrations should be prepared on separate sheets. *Tables* require a heading and figures a legend, also prepared on a separate sheet. The number of figures and tables should be limited and aim to illustrate the text. Figures are listed in the text as (fig. 1), tables as (table 1). Data already mentioned in the text need not be repeated in a table. Accordingly, numbers used in tables need not be repeated in the text.
For the reproduction of *illustrations*, only good drawings and original photographs can be accepted. On the back of each illustration, indicate its number, the author's name, and 'top' with a soft pencil. Electronically submitted b/w half-tone and color illustrations must have a final resolution of 300 dpi after scaling, line drawings one of 800–1200 dpi.
Color illustrations are reproduced at the author's expense. Each one is charged to the author at EUR 280,– + VAT as contribution to the additional reproduction and color printing costs.

References

The list of references should include only the publications cited in the text. References must be numbered sequentially in the order cited in the text. In the text identify references by Arabic numerals [in square brackets]. In each reference all authors should be named; the abbreviation 'et al.' is to be avoided. It is recommended to quote only articles already published or accepted for publication. Please avoid 'in preparation' or 'personal communication'. Authors are responsible for the accuracy and completeness of their references and for correct citation. Journal titles should be abbreviated according to the Index Medicus system (www.nlm.nih.gov). If a reference manager is used, the style «Pharmacology» or «Nephron» should be chosen.

Examples for references:

Papers published in periodicals:

1 Lelie PN, Cuypers HTM, van Drimmelen AAJ, Quint WGV: Quality assessment of hepatitis C virus nucleic acid amplification methods. An international proficiency study. Infusionsther Transfusionsmed 1998;25:102–110.

Papers published only with DOI numbers:

2 Theoharides TC, Boucher W, Spear K: Serum interleukin-6 reflects disease severity and osteoporosis in mastocytosis patients. Int Arch Allergy Immunol DOI: 10.1159/000063858.

Papers published in electronic format:

3 Black CA: Delayed type hypersensitivity: Current theories with a historic perspective. Dermatol Online J 1999;5:7. http://dermatology.dclib.org/DOJvol5num1.

Edited books:

4 Hardy WD Jr, Essex M: FeLV-induced feline acquired immune deficiency syndrome: A model for human AIDS; in Klein E (ed): Acquired Immunodeficiency Syndrome. Prog Allergy. Basel, Karger, 1986, vol 37, pp 353–376.

Monographs:

5 Schaefer UW, Beelen DW: Bone Marrow Transplantation, ed 2, revised. Basel, Karger, 1996.

Page Charges

There are no page charges for papers that do not exceed the allotted size (cf. types of papers). Each additional complete or partial page is charged to the author at 390,– EUR + VAT.

Galley Proofs

Unless indicated otherwise, galley proofs are sent to the corresponding author and should be returned with the least possible delay. Alterations made in galley proofs, other than the correction of printer's errors, are charged to the author. No page proofs are supplied.

Reprints

Order forms and a price list are sent with the galley proofs. Orders submitted after the issue is printed are subject to considerably higher prices.

KARGER

Fax +49 761 4 52 07 14
Information@Karger.de
www.karger.com

Accessible online at:
www.karger.com/tmh

Transfusion Medicine and Hemotherapy

Hinweise für Autoren

Transfus Med Hemother 2009;36

Einreichung von Manuskripten
Die Zeitschrift Transfusion Medicine and Hemotherapy ist ein Forum für alle Bereiche der Transfusionsmedizin, Hämostaseologie und Immunhämatologie. Veröffentlicht werden Arbeiten über wissenschaftliche, technische und administrative Fragen der Bluttransfusion, der Lagerung von Blutprodukten, der Infusionstherapie und über transfusionsmedizinische Aspekte der Transplantation. Alle Beiträge unterliegen einem unabhängigen Begutachtungsverfahren.

Manuskripte können online eingereicht werden: www.karger.com/tmh

Sollten Sie Probleme mit der Online-Einreichung haben oder es für notwendig halten, das Manuskript in nichtelektronischer Form einzureichen, senden Sie es bitte an:

S. Karger Verlag für Medizin und Naturwissenschaften GmbH
Dr. Sven Riestenpatt
Postfach
D-79095 Freiburg (Deutschland)
Tel. +49 761 45 20 722
Fax +49 761 45 20 714
E-mail s.riestenpatt@karger.de

Sprache
Alle Beiträge müssen in englischer Sprache (amerikanische oder britische Rechtschreibung) eingereicht werden.

Rubriken und Umfang
Die Manuskripte sollen in 1 1/2-zeiligem Abstand mit beidseitig je 3 cm Rand, Schrift 12 pt eingereicht werden.

Folgender Umfang sollte nicht überschritten werden:

	Druckseiten	Entspricht Manuskriptseiten*
Übersichtsarbeit, Originalarbeit	10	30
Kasuistik	3	9
Qualitätsmanagement, Klinische Information	5	15
Brief an die Herausgeber	2	6
Übrige Beiträge	2	6

* **einschließlich Zusammenfassung, Abbildungen, Tabellen und Literaturzitate**

Für Umfangsüberschreitungen wird dem Autor ein Mehrkostenanteil in Rechnung gestellt.

Bedingungen
Über die Annahme wissenschaftlicher Beiträge wird aufgrund mehrerer Gutachten entschieden (peer-review).
Der Verlag geht davon aus, dass eingereichte Manuskripte nicht gleichzeitig bei einem anderen Journal begutachtet werden. Die Einreichung eines Beitrags impliziert die Übertragung der Rechte auf den Verlag, falls das Manuskript angenommen wird.
Mit der Annahme des Manuskripts zur Publikation gehen alle Rechte auf den Verlag über. Die Übertragung der Nutzungsrechte bezieht sich sowohl auf alle Print- als auch auf elektronische Offline- und Onlinemedien unter Einschluss des Internets und von Datenbanken/Datenträgern aller Art. Ohne schriftliche Genehmigung des Verlages dürfen diese Publikationen oder Teile daraus nicht in andere Sprachen übersetzt oder in irgendeiner Form mit mechanischen oder elektronischen Mitteln (einschließlich Fotokopie, Tonaufnahme und Mikrofilm) reproduziert oder auf Datenträger oder einem Computersystem gespeichert werden. Es ist Sache des Autors, die Nachdruckerlaubnis für Abbildungen, Tabellen usw. aus anderen Publikationen zu beschaffen.
Alle Formen der Unterstützung, inklusive der durch Pharmaunternehmen, und potentielle Interessenskonflikte sollen in einem Begleitschreiben an den Herausgeber offen gelegt werden. Wird das Manuskript angenommen, so wird der Herausgeber mit dem Autor vereinbaren, inwieweit dies publiziert werden muss.
Typographische Gestaltung und redaktionelle Bearbeitung werden vom Verlag durchgeführt.

Ethische und rechtliche Voraussetzungen
Manuskripte, bei denen Untersuchungen an Probanden oder Patienten durchgeführt wurden, müssen die Erklärung enthalten, dass das Versuchsprotokoll von einer Ethikkommission genehmigt wurde und den ethischen Standards der Deklaration von Helsinki in ihrer erweiterten Form von 1975 und ihren Zusätzen von 1983, 1989 und 1996 [JAMA 1997;277:925–926] entspricht. Zugleich muss im Manuskripttext auf die Einwilligung der Versuchsperson nach Aufklärung hingewiesen werden. Angaben, die auf die Identität der Person schließen lassen, sind unzulässig.

Gliederung
Autorennamen und -adressen: Die vollständigen Autorennamen mit der jeweiligen Institutsangabe in der Landessprache der Autoren, die vollständige Postadresse des Korrespondenzautors, mit Telefon- und Faxnummer sowie E-Mail-Adresse sollen in einem separaten Dokument angegeben werden, um die anonyme Begutachtung sicherzustellen.

Titelseite: Die Titelseite muss den Titel und Kurztitel der Arbeit in Deutsch und Englisch enthalten.

Schlüsselwörter: Zu einer Arbeit gehören 3–5 **Schlüsselwörter** (Englisch und Deutsch), die möglichst der «Medical Subjects Heading List» des Index Medicus entnommen sein sollen.

Zusammenfassung: Jedes Manuskript muss eine englische und deutsche Zusammenfassung enthalten, die jeweils 200 Wörter nicht überschreiten. Zusammenfassungen von Originalarbeiten und Kasuistiken sind zu strukturieren in Hintergrund, Patienten und Methoden (oder Material und Methoden), Ergebnisse, Schlussfolgerungen.

Fußnoten: Fußnoten sollten nur in Tabellen verwendet werden.

Geschützte Produkt- bzw. Markennamen: Bei ihrem ersten Auftreten im Text müssen geschützte Produkt- und Markennamen mit einem hochgestellten ® bzw. ™ bezeichnet werden. Die Verantwortung für die korrekte Befolgung dieser Vorschrift liegt ausschließlich beim Autor.

Abbildungen und Tabellen: Abbildungen und Tabellen sollen auf separaten Seiten erstellt werden. *Tabellen* benötigen eine Überschrift und Abbildungen eine Legende. Die Anzahl der Abbildungen und Tabellen sollte limitiert sein, sie sollen den Text illustrieren. Hinweise auf Abbildungen und Tabellen erfolgen im Text mit (fig. 1) bzw. (table 1). Im Text genannte Informationen bedürfen keiner Wiederholung in einer Tabelle.
Für die Reproduktion von *Abbildungsvorlagen* sind nur gute Zeichnungen und Originalfotografien geeignet. Auf der Rückseite der Vorlage bitte den Namen des Autors, ein Titelstichwort, die Angabe, wo «oben» ist, sowie die Bildnummer mit einem weichen Bleistift vermerken. Elektronisch eingereichte Halbtonabbildungen (schwarzweiß oder farbig) müssen in der endgültigen Größe eine Auflösung von 300 dpi haben, Strichzeichnungen 800–1200 dpi.
Farbabbildungen sind möglich, dem Autor wird jedoch ein Reproduktions- und Druckkostenanteil von EUR 280,– + MWSt. pro Abbildung in Rechnung gestellt.

Referenzen
Das Literaturverzeichnis soll nur die im Text zitierten Publikationen enthalten. Die Literatur ist entsprechend der Reihenfolge des Auftretens im Text zu nummerieren. Die Referenzen werden als Zahlen [in eckigen Klammern] in den Text eingefügt. Bitte alle Autoren einer Arbeit angeben, die Abkürzung «et al.» ist zu vermeiden. Zitiert werden sollen nur Arbeiten, die entweder publiziert oder zur Publikation angenommen sind. Der Passus «in Vorbereitung» oder «persönliche Mitteilung» ist zu vermeiden. Die Autoren sind für eine korrekte und vollständige Zitierung der Referenzen verantwortlich. Die Abkürzung der Zeitschriftentitel erfolgt nach dem Index-Medicus-System (www.nlm.nih.gov). Wird ein Referenzmanager benutzt, sollte das Format «Pharmacology» oder «Nephron» gewählt werden.

Beispiele zur Abfassung von Literaturzitaten:

Zeitschriftenbeiträge:
1 Lelie PN, Cuypers HTM, van Drimmelen AAJ, Quint WGV: Quality assessment of hepatitis C virus nucleic acid amplification methods. An international proficiency study. Infusionsther Transfusionsmed 1998;25:102–110.

Artikel, die nur eine DOI-Nummer haben:
2 Theoharides TC, Boucher W, Spear K: Serum interleukin-6 reflects disease severity and osteoporosis in mastocytosis patients. Int Arch Allergy Immunol DOI: 10.1159/000063858.

Elektronisch publizierte Artikel:
3 Black CA: Delayed type hypersensitivity: Current theories with a historic perspective. Dermatol Online J 1999;5:7. http://dermatology.dclib.org/DOJvol5num1.

Bücher mit Herausgeber:
4 Hardy WD Jr, Essex M: FeLV-induced feline acquired immune deficiency syndrome: A model for human AIDS; in Klein E (ed): Acquired Immunodeficiency Syndrome. Prog Allergy. Basel, Karger, 1986, vol 37, pp 353–376.

Monographien:
5 Schaefer UW, Beelen DW: Bone Marrow Transplantation, ed 2, revised. Basel, Karger, 1996.

Kosten
Für Artikel mit maximal der vorgesehenen Seitenzahl werden keine Druckkosten erhoben (siehe Rubriken und Umfang). Jede weitere angefangene Druckseite wird dem Autor mit EUR 390,– + MWSt. pro Druckseite in Rechnung gestellt.

Druckfahnen
Falls nicht anders vereinbart werden die Druckfahnen dem Korrespondenzautor zugeschickt und sollen schnellstmöglich zurückgesandt werden. Änderungen in den Druckfahnen, die über die Korrektur von Satzfehlern hinausgehen, werden dem Autor in Rechnung gestellt. Es werden keine Umbruchabzüge versandt.

Sonderdrucke
Ein Formular und die Preisliste zur Sonderdruckbestellung werden mit den Druckfahnen versandt. Bestellungen, die nach Drucklegung bei uns eingehen, können nur zu wesentlich höheren Preisen ausgeführt werden.

KARGER
Fax +49 761 4 52 07 14
Information@Karger.de
www.karger.com

Accessible online at:
www.karger.com/tmh

Transfusion Medicine and Hemotherapy

Contents of Forthcoming Issues · Themenvorschau

Transfus Med Hemother 2009;36:100

KARGER
Fax +49 761 4 52 07 14
Information@Karger.de
www.karger.com

Accessible online at:
www.karger.com/tmh